THE AUTONOMIC
NERVOUS SYSTEM

THE AUTONOMIC NERVOUS SYSTEM

for students of Physiology
and of Pharmacology

J. HAROLD BURN

M.D., F.R.S., Hon. D.Sc., Yale;
Hon. M.D., Mainz; Dr. hon. causa. Paris.

Emeritus Professor of Pharmacology
University of Oxford

FOURTH EDITION

Blackwell Scientific Publications
Oxford and Edinburgh

© BLACKWELL SCIENTIFIC PUBLICATIONS 1963, 1965, 1968, 1971

SBN 632 08080 9

FIRST PUBLISHED 1963
SECOND EDITION 1965
THIRD EDITION 1968
FOURTH EDITION 1971

Printed in Great Britain by
Alden & Mowbray Ltd
at the Alden Press, Oxford
and bound at
the Kemp Hall Bindery

CONTENTS

PREFACE TO FOURTH EDITION

THE scope of this book has been considerably enlarged. It now includes a chapter on chemical transmission in the brain, dealing in particular with work on the nigro-striatal tract, and also with the identification of Gaba as an inhibitory transmitter by the discovery of bicucullin as an antagonist. The properties of 5-hydroxytryptamine, of the prostaglandins, of the polypeptides including angiotensin are discussed, and there is an account of transmission to the anterior pituitary gland. An account of Malik's work on the cholinergic link in the release of nor-adrenaline from sympathetic fibres is given together with the work of Ehinger and his colleagues and of de la Lande and his colleagues on the histological evidence which underlies the cholinergic link. I now consider the cholinergic link established.

Since the greater part of the book deals with substances present in the body, it concerns physiologists as much as pharmacologists and is of importance to those in clinical work, especially in clinical research. I am indebted to Dr. K. U. Malik for permission to include Figs. 17.1, 17.2, 17.3, 17.4, 17.5, 17.6 and 17.7 and to the Editor of Circulation Research for permission to include the first four of these. I am indebted to Prof. M. J. Rand and to the Editor of *Nature* for permission to include Fig. 19.1 and finally I am indebted to Dr. Ehinger and to the Editor of *Z. Zellforschung* for permission to include Fig. 21.1.

August 1970   J. H. BURN

CHAPTER I

EARLY WORK ON ACETYLCHOLINE

The autonomic system and chemical transmission. In 1898 Langley wrote 'I propose the term "autonomic nervous system", for the sympathetic system and the allied nervous system of the cranial and sacral nerves, and for the local nervous system of the gut'. The term did not, however, gain general acceptance at first, and Gaskell called it 'The involuntary nervous system' in his book published in 1916. However, the passage of time has favoured Langley and to-day the autonomic nerves are generally regarded as the motor nerves of the sympathetic and parasympathetic systems.

The involuntary reflex arcs. Gaskell made the understanding of the anatomy of the autonomic nerves much easier by suggesting that they could be considered in terms of reflex arcs. He took as the model reflex arc an arc consisting of three neurones. The first neurone was a sensory or receptor neurone, beginning in the skin and ending in the posterior horn of the spinal cord. Its cell station was in the posterior root ganglion. The second neurone was a connector neurone, beginning from a cell in the posterior horn and ending in the anterior horn. The third neurone was a motor or excitor neurone, beginning from a cell in the anterior horn and proceeding to a skeletal muscle in the periphery (see Fig. 1.1).

Gaskell then described the sympathetic reflex arc as a variant of this. The sympathetic reflex arc had the same three components. There was a sensory or receptor fibre which began in the skin and ended, not in the posterior horn, but in the lateral horn of the spinal cord, thus proceeding rather further. The connector fibre began from a cell in the lateral horn, and travelled out of the anterior horn as a white ramus communicans until it

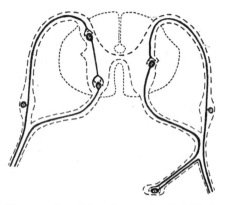

FIG. 1.1. Gaskell's conception of the reflex arc. On the left is shown the voluntary reflex arc consisting of sensory fibre, connector fibre and motor fibre. On the right the sympathetic reflex arc consisting of the same three fibres. The connector fibre runs out of the spinal cord entering a sympathetic ganglion as a preganglionic fibre. The motor fibre begins in the sympathetic ganglion as a postganglionic fibre.

reached a sympathetic ganglion. In the ganglion the connector fibre ended and formed a synapse around the cell of the excitor or motor fibre, the axon of which left the ganglion and proceeded as a grey ramus communicans to a mixed spinal nerve, finally to reach an end organ such as the wall of a blood vessel. Thus the essential difference between the ordinary reflex arc and the sympathetic reflex arc was that the synapse between the connector and the excitor fibre was in the anterior horn for the former, but had moved out of the spinal cord to a sympathetic ganglion for the latter.

The parasympathetic reflex arc was another variant. There were again the three components. The sensory or receptor fibre began in the periphery and (taking the vagus as an example) ran upwards, having its cell station in the nodose ganglion (which corresponds to an ordinary posterior root ganglion) and terminating in the medulla around the dorsal nucleus of the vagus. Thus the dorsal nucleus of the vagus formed the beginning of the connector fibre, and the connector fibre then ran out of the medulla and continued all the way to the end organ which might be the heart or the intestine. Having reached the heart, the connector fibres formed a synapse around cells which gave rise to extremely short excitor fibres; they terminated almost as soon as they began. These cells, which give rise to extremely short excitor fibres are, in the intestine, the cells of Auerbach's plexus (see Fig. 1.2).

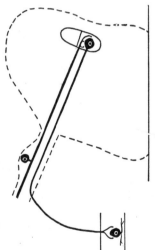

FIG. 1.2. This shows Gaskell's conception of the parasympathetic reflex arc. The sensory fibre ends in the dorsal nucleus of the vagus in the medulla. The connector fibre begins in this nucleus, and travels out from the central nervous system to the end organ (the heart or the intestine) where it terminates around the motor fibre which begins and ends at once. The motor fibre is, for example, a cell of Auerbach's plexus.

Function of the autonomic systems. Both the sympathetic and parasympathetic systems are alike in differing from the voluntary nervous system in one respect. The involuntary systems to some extent work as a whole; when one part of the sympathetic system is active, other parts are also active.

The sympathetic system is responsible for the changes seen in fear, in anger, and in other strong emotions. As Cannon has described, the sympathetic system prepares the animal for fight or for flight. The heart increases in rate and in force of beat. The blood vessels constrict, in particular those to the skin and the viscera. The pupils of the eyes dilate, the bronchioles dilate, the blood sugar rises and the hair is erected.

The parasympathetic system is active during digestion and sleep. The picture has been presented of parasympathetic activity in an old man sleeping after dinner. His heart rate is slow, his breathing noisy because of brochial constriction, his pupils are small, drops of saliva may run out of the corner of his mouth. A stethoscope applied to his abdomen will reveal much intestinal activity.

The concept of chemical transmission. The account which follows will describe the evidence that the effects of the sympathetic system are in the main exerted by the release of noradrenaline (norepinephrine) at the terminations of the postganglionic fibres, and that the effects of the parasympathetic system are exerted by the release of acetylcholine.

The concept of chemical transmission of nerve impulses appears to have arisen from the studies of the early pharmacologists on the action of poisonous substances found in plants, to discover what effects they produced in the body. An alkaloid obtained from *Amanita muscaria*, a toadstool which attracted flies, was muscarine, and muscarine was found to have many effects in the body like those of parasympathetic stimulation. The question appears to have been asked whether parasympathetic nerves might produce their effects by liberating muscarine.

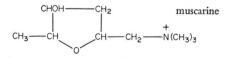

About the sympathetic system there is no doubt. When the substance called by Abel epinephrin, and called by Takamine adrenalin, was obtained in pure form by Takamine from the adrenal medulla, examination of its effects in the body suggested to Elliott that sympathetic postganglionic fibres might exert their action by releasing it.

The properties of acetylcholine. Strecker in 1849 gave the name choline to a base he found present in pig bile. In 1899 Reid Hunt found it in the adrenal gland, and in 1911 Hunt and Taveau discovered that the acetic ester of choline, acetylcholine, was extremely powerful in causing a fall of blood pressure in the cat. An examination of this substance was made by Dale as the result of what seemed to be an accident. Dale was testing the effect of an extract of ergot, and observed that when it was injected into a cat, the heart was arrested and the blood pressure fell to zero. Since the injection of an extract of ergot had not previously had this effect, Dale concluded that he had killed the cat by blowing air into its vein. However, after a minute or two the blood pressure recovered, and Dale then satisfied himself that this extract of ergot contained a highly active substance not normally present. Its behaviour suggested that it might be muscarine. His colleague Ewins then attempted to isolate the substance, and found that, unlike muscarine, it was very unstable. Dale then remembered the result of Hunt and Taveau, and asked Ewins to synthesize acetylcholine in order that it might be compared with the extract of ergot. Proof was obtained that acetylcholine was present in the extract.

Since choline esters had been variously reported as causing a fall of blood pressure and also a rise of blood pressure, Dale [1] examined the cardiovascular action of acetylcholine. He found that very small amounts, 2 μg. or less, caused a fall of blood pressure on intravenous injection, while larger amounts, 40 μg., caused great slowing of the heart as well. The fall of blood

5

pressure caused by amounts such as 2 µg. was due to a vasodilator action on the vessel wall, for it was seen when an ear of a rabbit removed after death was perfused with Ringer's solution through the central artery. When acetylcholine was injected into the perfusing fluid, the vessels dilated, and the outflow from the ear increased. These properties, the vasodilatation and cardiac inhibition, resembled those of muscarine, and like the properties of muscarine they were abolished by atropine.

The belladonna alkaloids. There are two alkaloids, atropine and hyoscine, which are obtained from the plants *Atropa bella-donna*, *Hyoscyamus niger* and *Datura stramonium*. When acetyl-choline acts on the heart, causing slowing of the rate or complete arrest, it is said to do so by forming a combination with 'recep-tors', and when the combination is formed, slowing of the rate results. Atropine, or hyoscine, is said to have an affinity for the same receptors, with the difference that when atropine is given, the union between it and the receptors persists for a long time. So long as atropine remains attached to the receptors, acetyl-choline is unable to act.

The nicotine-like action of acetylcholine. Because the action of acetylcholine on the heart and blood vessels in small amounts was like that of muscarine and was abolished by atropine, Dale described these actions as muscarine-like. He then observed that acetylcholine had other actions in the presence of atropine which were exerted when the doses were sufficiently large. If the dose was raised from 2 µg. to 2 mg., that is one thousand times, then the injection of acetylcholine caused a rise of blood pressure. The rise showed a step on its upward course. There was a steep initial rise, then a pause, and a further pro-longed rise attended by great quickening of the heart. The rise in general resembled the rise when nicotine was injected; it was due to stimulation of the sympathetic ganglion in the first place:

6

this resulted in a discharge of impulses along postganglionic fibres to the blood vessels, causing them to constrict. The rise was due in the second place to a discharge of adrenaline (epinephrine) from the medulla of the adrenal glands; this caused

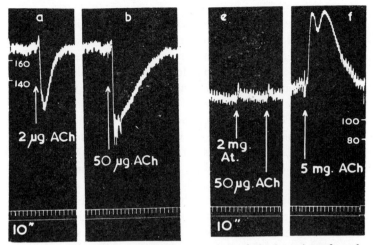

FIG. 1.3. Dale's demonstration of the muscarine and nicotine actions of acetylcholine on the blood pressure of the cat. In (a) is shown the depressor action of 2μg. acetylcholine injected intravenously. This fall of pressure is due to vasodilatation. In (b) is shown the depressor action of 50μg. acetylcholine which causes an abrupt drop due to slowing of the heart, as well as to vasodilatation. The effects in (a) and (b) are muscarine like. In (e) 2mg. atropine was injected, and in its presence 50μg. acetylcholine had no effect. In (f) 5mg. acetylcholine caused a rise of blood pressure due first to stimulation of sympathetic ganglia, and second to stimulation of the adrenal medulla.

further vasoconstriction and great acceleration of the heart (see Fig. 1.3).

When repeated injections of nicotine are made, the rise of blood pressure which they cause declines in size, and is finally absent. This is because an excess of nicotine paralyses the structures which it at first stimulates. When paralysis to nicotine

7

has been produced, acetylcholine can then no longer cause a rise of blood pressure.

Dale therefore described acetylcholine as possessing not only muscarine-like properties, but also nicotine-like properties which could be seen when the muscarine-like properties were abolished by atropine.

The distinction between properties of acetylcholine which are muscarine-like and abolished by atropine, and those which are nicotine-like and seen in the presence of atropine, has proved very useful. However it has led to the conception that any tissue on which acetylcholine acts must have either the one kind of receptor or the other, but not both. Thus it was thought that the receptors on which acetylcholine acted to stimulate ganglia were nicotinic receptors. It was therefore a surprise when Ambache, Perry and Robertson [268] found in 1956 that when the superior cervical ganglion was perfused, muscarine itself would cause stimulation, and this action was abolished by atropine. They also showed that atropine had some effect in depressing the response of the ganglion to acetylcholine. Thus it appeared that the ganglion had both muscarinic and nicotinic receptors for acetylcholine.

Another example is the sympathetic postganglionic fibre which may be blocked at its termination by acetylcholine [266]. This block is removed by atropine, but a similar block caused by DMPP (dimethylphenyl piperazinium) is not removed by atropine [267].

Loewi's demonstration of chemical transmission. In 1921 Otto Loewi [2] published an account of his demonstration of humoral or chemical transmission. This means the transmission of a nerve impulse through the release of a chemical substance which, like a drug, produces the physiological effect.

The experiment was done very simply, and Loewi has described how the idea occurred to him when in bed, and how he went at once to the laboratory to carry it out. He used the heart of the frog, inserting a Straub cannula through the bulbus aortae into the ventricle. The cannula consisted of a small glass tube with a nozzle to fit into the ventricle. The ventricle was filled with frog Ringer, and, at each contraction, the ventricle drove the Ringer up the cannula. When the ventricle relaxed, the Ringer fell back into the ventricle again. Thus the fluid was not changed, and successive contractions drove the same fluid out of the ventricle, allowing it to return again during relaxation. He dissected the vagal-sympathetic trunk, and placed it upon electrodes, so that he could stimulate it. Stimulation caused arrest of the heart, but the beats were resumed soon after stimulation stopped. Loewi then carried out his experiment. He stimulated the vagus and stopped the heart. Then with a pipette he removed the Ringer's solution from the arrested ventricle, and replaced it with fresh Ringer. The heart resumed its beats. A minute or so later, he took out the fresh Ringer, and replaced the Ringer withdrawn during the arrest. Replacing this Ringer caused the beat to be arrested again. Thus Loewi demonstrated that when the nerve was stimulated, a substance was released into the cavity of the ventricle and was retained in the fluid in the ventricle. This fluid, when removed, could cause arrest of the heart at another time, or could cause the arrest of another heart when introduced into the ventricle. He called the unknown substance 'vagusstoff'.

Loewi observed that the action of vagusstoff was abolished by atropine. When he treated the frog heart with atropine, stimulation of the vagus-sympathetic trunk no longer caused inhibition of the heart, but caused acceleration instead. (This acceleration was seen much better in the heart of the toad than in the heart of the frog.) He therefore concluded that when he had given atropine, he had prevented the action of vagusstoff, but had unmasked the action of 'acceleransstoff', liberated by the sympathetic fibres. Thus he had demonstrated not only that the parasympathetic nerves transmitted their impulses chemically, but that the sympathetic fibres did so too.

The action of eserine. The identity of vagusstoff was not proved for some years. It was clear that it behaved like an unstable ester of choline, such as acetylcholine, but while choline was known to be present in the animal body, acetylcholine was not.

Help in the identification of vagusstoff came from the use of eserine (also called physostigmine) which is an alkaloid obtained from the Calabar bean. This is a black bean, about the size of an olive, which had long been used in trials by ordeal in the area of the delta of the Niger. Workers as far back as 1905 had shown that small doses of eserine increased the effectiveness of parasympathetic impulses. For example, eserine, put within the eyelid in the conjunctival sac, increased the effect of stimulating the third nerve in causing constriction of the pupil. Reid Hunt showed in 1918 that eserine increased the effects of acetylcholine, both the muscarine-like effects, and the nicotine-like effects. In the same year Fühner [3] found that eserine greatly increased the action of acetylcholine in causing contraction of the isolated muscle of the leech. Eserine did not increase the action of pilocarpine or of choline, but increased the action of acetylcholine one million times. Fühner suggested that the effect of eserine was to inhibit hydrolysis of acetylcholine by the tissue. In the course of hydrolysis acetylcholine is broken down to choline and acetic acid.

$$\text{Acetylcholine} \quad (CH_3)_3 \cdot \overset{+}{N} \cdot CH_2 \cdot CH_2 \cdot O \cdot CO \cdot CH_3$$

$$\text{Choline} \quad (CH_3)_3 \cdot \overset{+}{N} \cdot CH_2 \cdot CH_2 \cdot OH$$

Loewi and Navratil [4] in 1926 therefore applied eserine to the identification of 'vagusstoff'. They found that eserine prolonged the effect of stimulating the vagus in inhibiting the beat of the frog heart. They also found that it prolonged the action of the vagusstoff itself. It prolonged the action of acetylcholine on the heart, but not that of muscarine or of choline. Next they investigated the action of eserine on the enzyme in the muscle of the frog heart which destroys both vagusstoff and acetylcholine. They found that eserine inhibited the destruction of both. All their results pointed to vagusstoff being acetylcholine.

The enzyme in the body which splits acetylcholine by hydrolysis is now known as cholinesterase. Its action is inhibited by eserine and by other 'anticholinesterases', such as neostigmine which is a substance made in the laboratory.

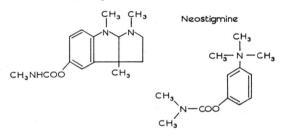

CHAPTER 2

THE GENERAL DEMONSTRATION
OF CHEMICAL TRANSMISSION

ABOUT the same time that Loewi and Navratil were demonstrating the relation between acetylcholine and vagusstoff, Dale
and Gasser [5] were contributing to another chapter which had
been begun as early as 1863. It concerned curious observations
made by several workers on the behaviour of denervated skeletal
muscle.

For the moment the work of Böhm (1908) will serve as the
starting point, for he showed that choline caused a contraction
of the rectus abdominis muscle of the frog when removed from
the body and tested as an isolated preparation. This contraction
occurred in the normal muscle of the frog, but not in normal
mammalian muscle. Later acetylcholine was observed to be
more active than choline on frog muscle, and then in 1922 it
was discovered that acetylcholine would cause contraction of
mammalian muscle in quite small amounts if the muscle had
first been denervated. Until that time it was not known that
acetylcholine had an action on mammalian skeletal muscle. The
work of Dale and Gasser confirmed and greatly clarified the
position. They showed that the skeletal muscle of the dog and
the cat, from six to seven days after section of the motor nerves,
became sensitive to acetylcholine, and contracted in response to
it. This action of acetylcholine was not abolished by atropine
and was not a muscarine-like property, but a nicotine-like
property of acetylcholine. The property was in fact shared by
nicotine, and by several other substances which had a nicotine-
like action in other directions. Such substances were cytisine

(the alkaloid present in laburnum seeds), tetramethylammonium, and the nitrous ester of choline. On the other hand, muscarine and pilocarpine, the actions of which were abolished by atropine, did not cause contraction of denervated skeletal muscle. Nor did histamine.

Thus acetylcholine was shown to be concerned in three physiological situations. It had effects like those of the parasympathetic system which were abolished by atropine. It had other effects which were not abolished by atropine, and these were of two kinds. First it caused stimulation of all autonomic ganglia and of the adrenal medulla, and second it caused stimulation of denervated skeletal muscle.

The presence of acetylcholine in the body. In 1929 the discovery was made by Dale and Dudley [6] that acetylcholine was present in the body. They were able to isolate it from the spleen of the horse and to identify it. Just as the isolation of adrenaline from the adrenal medulla was followed by progress in knowledge of the sympathetic system, so the isolation of acetylcholine was followed by great progress in the fields where acetylcholine played a part.

Curious reactions of denervated muscle. The early work already mentioned was carried out in 1863 by two French workers, Vulpian and Philippeaux. They showed that when the hypoglossal nerve, which is a motor nerve to the tongue, was divided and allowed to degenerate, the muscles of the tongue acquired a new type of sensitiveness, for they went into a state of contracture as a result of stimulation of the chorda tympani. The chorda tympani is a secretory nerve to the submaxillary gland, a parasympathetic nerve causing a flow of saliva. It was known since 1883 that nicotine would cause contracture of the denervated tongue, and in 1923 it was shown that acetylcholine would cause it to contract as well.

The stage was thus set for reaching the conclusion that the parasympathetic nerve, the chorda tympani, released acetylcholine when stimulated, and that this acetylcholine was responsible for the contracture of the denervated tongue, the muscles of which were very sensitive to its action because they were denervated. Dale and Gaddum [7] studied the contracture of the tongue in response to stimulation of the chorda, and concluded that the 'direct effect of the nerve impulses was the liberation at their peripheral endings in relation to the blood vessels of a labile diffusible substance which stimulates contracture in the sensitized muscle'. By using eserine they obtained strong support for the view that this substance was acetylcholine. Thus they were able to observe contractures of the tongue in three ways: (a) by the stimulation of the chorda tympani, (b) by the injection of acetylcholine, and (c) by the injection of tetramethylammonium which is a substance having a nicotine-like action. This substance is not hydrolyzed by the esterase which destroys acetylcholine and which is inhibited by eserine. When eserine was injected they observed that the contractures of the tongue produced by stimulation of the chorda and by injection of acetylcholine were greatly increased, while the contraction produced by injection of tetramethylammonium was unchanged.

Their evidence thus indicated that stimulation of the chorda tympani, a mammalian parasympathetic nerve, like stimulation of the vagus in the frog, produced its effect by liberating acetylcholine.

The Rogowicz phenomenon. Another very curious phenomenon observed in early days was recorded by Rogowicz in 1885. He cut the facial nerve in the dog and allowed it to degenerate. He then found that the muscles moving the lips of the dog acquired a new power of contracting in response to stimulation of the cervical sympathetic nerve. This was again a situation in which denervated skeletal muscles responded by contracture to the stimulation of an autonomic nerve. But this time the autonomic nerve was a sympathetic nerve, and on the assumption that a sympathetic nerve releases a chemical substance, the substance was commonly believed to be adrenaline (epinephrine) or a close relative of it. The substance was not expected to be acetylcholine. However, Euler and Gaddum [8], who investigated the phenomenon in 1931, came to the conclusion that stimulation of the sympathetic in fact released acetylcholine, and thus, although the fibres were anatomically sympathetic, they were pharmacologically parasympathetic. Their evidence again turned on the use of eserine.

The result was not so surprising as it may sound, because it had been shown by Dastre and Morat in 1880 that stimulation of the sympathetic which, of course, usually produces pallor in superficial areas, often produced blushing or dilatation in the area of the dog's lips. It appeared that there were special vasodilator fibres in the sympathetic supply to this region, and that the vasodilatation was due to the release of acetylcholine. It is likely that blushing in man is also caused by sympathetic impulses which release acetylcholine.

The splanchnic nerves and the adrenal medulla. In the year 1933 two important papers appeared which served as a prelude to the study of the transmission of impulses through ganglia, the transmission that is of the nerve impulse from the preganglionic to the postganglionic fibre. One concerned the mechanism of the release of adrenaline from the adrenal medulla when the splanchnic nerve was stimulated. The splanchnic nerve is preganglionic, and the cells of the adrenal medulla which receive impulses from this nerve are regarded as equivalent to postganglionic fibres.

Feldberg and Minz [9] carried out experiments because of the fact that acetylcholine was known to liberate adrenaline from the adrenal medulla. This led them to wonder if the splanchnic nerves liberated acetylcholine, and whether it was the acetylcholine so liberated which in turn liberated adrenaline.

A lumbar vein passes over the left adrenal on its way to the vena cava, and the blood leaving the adrenal gland enters this vein. They tied a cannula in the lumbar vein so that they could collect the adrenal blood, and then they stimulated the splanchnic nerve. They gave eserine to the dog beforehand, so that any acetylcholine liberated would not be destroyed. They tested the blood from the adrenal vein both before and during stimulation. One test was made on the muscle of the leech previously suspended in Ringer's solution containing eserine. Blood taken before stimulation did not make the leech muscle contract, while blood taken during stimulation caused a large contraction. Thus Feldberg and Minz made use of Fühner's discovery that the leech muscle when treated with eserine was extremely sensitive to the action of acetylcholine. Other tests were made on the blood pressure of the cat, and these confirmed the tests on the leech in showing that acetylcholine was liberated when the splanchnic nerve was stimulated.

The second paper was written by Chang and Gaddum [10].

Its object was twofold. First to measure the amounts of acetylcholine present in different tissues of the body. In the course of this work they found that a fair amount of acetylcholine was present in the sympathetic chain, and this led them to ask whether acetylcholine might act as a transmitter in sympathetic ganglia. The second object of the paper was to show how a fluid containing a substance with properties resembling those of acetylcholine could be examined so as to make certain that the substance present was acetylcholine and not another ester of choline. They accomplished this by the method of parallel quantitative tests on different objects. They examined six esters of choline and also choline itself, comparing them with acetylcholine by five different tests. These tests are shown in Table 2. Thus propionylcholine when compared with acetylcholine was found to have a quite different relationship on the rabbit intestine from that on the frog rectus. When acetylcholine was given the value 100, propionylcholine had the value 3·0 on the rabbit intestine, but it had the value 550·0 on the frog rectus. Chang and Gaddum therefore proposed that in testing for the presence of acetylcholine in any fluid by comparison with a known solution of acetylcholine, the tests should be made on two or three organs, in order to see if the same equivalence was obtained on each. Only if the same equivalence was found could the substance in the fluid be said to be acetylcholine. This was an important principle.

The heart-lung preparation. As a result of Hitler's accession to power in 1933, Feldberg left Germany in that year to join Dale's laboratory in London. Before doing so, however, he showed together with Krayer [11] that the transmission of vagal impulses to the mammalian heart was effected by acetylcholine, as Loewi had shown in the frog heart. They used the Starling heart-lung preparation of the dog, and collected blood from the coronary sinus. The preparation was eserinized. Blood samples were tested on the leech. They observed that samples collected before vagal stimulation did not cause contraction of the leech muscle. Samples collected during vagal stimulation, however, did so.

Transmission in the sympathetic ganglion. In 1933 the Russian physiologist Kibjakow [12] published an elegant method of perfusing the superior cervical ganglion of the cat with a modified Ringer's solution. The fluid which left the ganglion in the venous effluent could be collected and tested for the presence of active substances. The perfused ganglion transmitted impulses, and stimulation of the preganglionic fibres caused contraction of the nictitating membrane. Feldberg and Gaddum [13] used this preparation to see if preganglionic stimulation led to the appearance of acetylcholine in the venous effluent. Feldberg was led to do this by his observation that splanchnic stimulation caused acetylcholine to appear in the adrenal vein, and Gaddum was led to do it by his observation that the tissue of the sympathetic chain contained acetylcholine.

TABLE 2.1

Results of parallel quantitative assays of choline esters in terms of acetylcholine, which was given the value 100.

(Chang and Gaddum, 1933.)

| Substances | Rabbit | | Frog Rectus | | Leech eserinized |
	Intestine	Blood pressure	Normal	Eserinized	
Choline	0·075	0·005	0·14	0·035	0·015
Propionylcholine	3·0	4·0	550·0	450·0	45·0
Butyrylcholine	0·24	0	90·0	115·0	90·0
Valerylcholine	0·2	0	25·0	30·0	0·9
Glycollylcholine	0·22	0·25	1·2	1·0	0·13
*Pyruvylcholine	14·0	10·0	13·0	13·0	16·0
Carbaminoylcholine	80·0	15·0	18·0	5·0	12·0

* See Gill, E. W., Parsons, J. A., and Paton, W. D. M. (1961) *J. Physiol.* (Lond.) **157**, 31P.

They observed that when the perfusion fluid contained eserine, then the venous effluent from the ganglion, collected during preganglionic stimulation, had three effects which indicated the presence of a substance like acetylcholine. These were contraction of the leech muscle, slowing of the rate of beating of the isolated auricle of the rabbit, and diminution of the amplitude of contraction of the heart of the frog. They proceeded to prove that this substance must be acetylcholine by showing that when the venous effluent collected during preganglionic stimulation was compared with a known solution of acetylcholine, its equivalence was the same (*a*) when tested on the frog heart and on the leech, and, in other experiments (*b*) when tested on the frog rectus and on the cat's blood pressure. The concentration of acetylcholine which they measured in the venous effluent was in one experiment between 15 and 30 μg. per litre, and in another between 30 and 50 μg. per litre. The leech preparations were in some cases so sensitive that they would have detected 1·5 μg. per litre, but in the fluid collected when there was no stimulation, not even this small amount of acetylcholine was present. The observations were consistent with the conclusion that preganglionic stimulation liberated acetylcholine. When acetylcholine was injected into the perfusing fluid without stimulation of the preganglionic fibres, action potentials could be picked up from the postganglionic fibres. Thus the evidence showed that preganglionic stimulation liberated acetylcholine, and that acetylcholine could stimulate the ganglion cells to discharge impulses along the postganglionic fibres.

The fibres to the sweat glands. The cat has long been known to sweat on the pads of its feet, and the soft pads of the young cat are specially suited to the study of sweating. The innervation of the sweat glands is sympathetic, and it has therefore been anomalous that sweating can no longer be seen if atropine is injected. Atropine does not prevent other sympathetic effects. Dale and Feldberg [14] examined the innervation of the sweat glands, and observed that the sympathetic fibres on stimulation liberated acetylcholine. The action of the fibres was not only abolished by atropine, but before atropine was given the action was increased by eserine. When the vessels of the foot were perfused with Ringer's solution containing eserine, stimulation of the sympathetic fibres caused the appearance of acetylcholine in the venous outflow.

The fact that fibres belonging to the sympathetic system were observed to release, not an adrenaline-like substance, but acetylcholine, led Dale to introduce the new terms. He proposed that nerve fibres which release an adrenaline-like substance should be called adrenergic fibres, and that fibres which release acetyl-choline should be called cholinergic fibres, fibres, that is to say, which work by liberating acetylcholine. Thus sympathetic fibres to the blood vessels were adrenergic, while those to the sweat glands were cholinergic.

The motor fibres to skeletal muscles. The observation that skeletal muscle when denervated was extremely sensitive to acetylcholine made it likely that acetylcholine might play a role in the transmission of impulses from motor nerves also. Dale, Feldberg and Vogt [15] showed that this was true. They tested several preparations. First they perfused the tongue of the cat. They used animals in which the superior cervical ganglia were removed two weeks previously in order to ensure degeneration of sympathetic fibres. They stimulated the hypoglossal nerve to the tongue when perfused with Ringer's solution containing eserine, and collected the fluid leaving the veins. They tested it on the leech and on the blood pressure of the cat, and observed that it contained acetylcholine. They made similar experiments perfusing the gastrocnemius muscles of cats and of dogs, when they stimulated the motor roots.

The evidence that motor nerves to skeletal muscle were cholinergic and released acetylcholine served to underline the curious fact that acetylcholine when injected into the blood stream did not cause muscle contractions. However, Brown, Dale and Feldberg [16] showed that if acetylcholine was injected into an artery at the point of entry into a muscle, then a contraction of the muscle was observed. They called this injection a 'close-arterial' injection.

Transmission in the spinal cord. The bulk of the work which has been described was published during the years 1934 to 1936. Five years later it was shown that transmission in some parts of the spinal cord was effected by acetylcholine. Bülbring and

Burn [17] made a preparation in which the lower half of the spinal cord of a dog was perfused by one circulation of blood, while the muscles of one hind leg were perfused by a second circulation of blood. They were able to show that amounts of acetylcholine as small as 1 μg., when injected into the spinal cord circulation following a small dose of eserine, would cause a series of contractions of the anterior tibialis muscle. They were also able to show that when the flexor reflex was recorded, the injection of eserine into the circulation through the spinal cord increased the size of the reflex contraction. Finally they were able to show that when the spinal cord was perfused by a Ringer's solution containing eserine, stimulation of the central end of the sciatic nerve caused the appearance of acetylcholine in the venous outflow from the spinal cord.

Potentiating effect of adrenaline. In the experiments described, adrenaline was found to have a potentiating action. Thus when an injection of acetylcholine into the blood perfusing the spinal chord failed to cause contractions in the anterior tibial muscle, the same dose became effective during the infusion of adrenaline into the spinal cord. Moreover, when the flexor reflex was elicited, the reflex was small; it was however very greatly increased by a slow infusion of adrenaline into the spinal cord. Finally, when the flexor reflex was elicited it was unaffected by the injection of neostigmine into the cord. However, during an infusion of adrenaline into the cord, the injection of neostigmine increased the reflex by 50 per cent [17].

These observations are probably of considerable importance because they indicate the part which may be played by adrenaline not only in the spinal cord but also in the brain. The effect of acetylcholine may be profoundly influenced by the concentration of adrenaline in the neighbourhood.

CHAPTER 3

TRANSMISSION THROUGH
THE GANGLION

Liberation of acetylcholine. As has already been described, when the superior cervical ganglion of the cat is perfused with the modified Ringer's solution described as Locke's solution, and when the perfusing fluid contains eserine to inhibit the action of cholinesterase, then stimulation of the preganglionic fibres results in the appearance of acetylcholine in the fluid leaving the ganglion. Several factors have been shown to modify the release of acetylcholine.

When the preganglionic fibres are stimulated at regular intervals, the amount of acetylcholine released in the perfusate rapidly declines. Birks and MacIntosh [20] have shown that this is because of deficiency of choline. When choline is added to the fluid perfusing the ganglion, the amount of acetylcholine liberated by successive periods of stimulation does not decline and remains constant at the initial high level.

If the ganglion is perfused with plasma and not with Locke's solution, the decline in acetylcholine output does not occur, because plasma contains sufficient choline.

Effect of physostigmine on transmission. The transmission of preganglionic impulses to the postganglionic fibre is not increased by physostigmine (eserine) when the stimuli applied to the preganglionic fibres are maximal. Because he failed to observe an increase to a single preganglionic volley, Eccles was led to doubt whether acetylcholine was in fact the ganglionic transmitter. However, Feldberg and Vartiainen [112] showed that when the stimuli were submaximal, physostigmine then improved transmission.

The Hemicholiniums. A series of compounds which have an unusual toxicity were described by Schueler [18]. These compounds contain choline incorporated into a six-membered ring through hemi-acetal formation. One of them has the formula

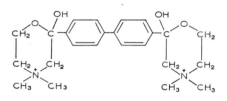

In the animal they cause paralysis of respiration, and when the dose is not very large the paralysis can be prevented by giving choline or eserine. MacIntosh, Birks and Sastry [19] thought that hemicholinium might specifically prevent the synthesis of acetylcholine, and were able to show that the compound just mentioned did so.

They prepared the superior cervical ganglion for perfusion, using plasma (and not Locke's solution) containing eserine. They found that when hemicholinium was added to the perfusion fluid, the rate at which acetylcholine was released into the perfusion fluid by stimulating the preganglionic fibres was unaffected when the stimulation lasted for 1–2 min. only. However, with longer stimulation, the rate of release of acetylcholine rapidly declined and the ganglion lost its ability to transmit impulses, and also its store of preformed acetylcholine. MacIntosh and his colleagues showed that the amount of acetylcholine synthesized in 1 hour by the ganglion was reduced from 1·21 μg. to 0·1 μg. when hemicholinium was present. They further made the very important observation that the effects of hemicholinium could be antagonized by raising the choline concentration of the plasma used for perfusion. Similar results were obtained with hemicholinium in minced mouse brain. Hemicholinium diminished the synthesis of acetylcholine by 75 per cent, while choline increased the synthesis and reversed the inhibitory effect of hemicholinium. The authors considered that hemicholinium might compete with choline for transport by a specific carrier mechanism to sites within the neurones where the acetylation of choline took place.

The site of acetylcholinesterase. The following consideration of ganglionic transmission has been presented by Koelle [224]. The neuronal acetylcholinesterase (AChE) in the superior cervical ganglion of the cat has been shown to be separated by the cell membrane into an external fraction and an internal fraction. Transmission is effected by inhibition of only the former. Thus the functional AChE is entirely presynaptic, and not as at the neuromuscular junction mostly post-synaptic. This suggests that AChE serves different primary functions at the two sites. Volle has determined the mean threshold dose of carbamyl-choline and of acetylcholine for producing postganglionic activation both in normal cats and in cats in which the pre-ganglionic fibres had been cut and had degenerated. Since denervation generally reduces the threshold dose, it was surprising to find that the threshold dose for carbamylcholine was raised about 30 times. When the AChE was inactivated by the anti-cholinesterase dyflos (see p. 34) then the threshold dose for acetylcholine was also found to be raised. It was 5 times as great for a denervated ganglion as for a normal ganglion. Koelle therefore suggests that the threshold dose of acetylcholine and carbamylcholine in normal cats activates only presynaptic terminals. These then liberate acetylcholine immediately adjacent to post-synaptic receptor sites, which in turn activate ganglion cells. Following denervation the higher thresholds represent the amounts required for direct excitation of ganglion cells. He suggests that the primary function of the presynaptic AChE is to limit the effect of the acetylcholine liberated to the presynaptic terminals themselves.

Ganglion stimulants and blocking agents. There are many substances which stimulate ganglia, and which also block transmission of impulses arriving at the preganglionic terminations. Perhaps the best-known substance is nicotine. When nicotine first reaches ganglion cells it causes stimulation, but after repeated application it no longer stimulates but causes block. There are many other substances which behave in this way, which are mostly 'onium' compounds, having a group similar to trimethylammonium, $-\overset{+}{N}(CH_3)_3$, in the molecule. One of the first of these to be studied was tetramethylammonium; this stimulates like nicotine and then on repetition the stimulant action declines until it is no longer seen.

Paton's rate theory of drug action. The action of these compounds has been studied by Paton [117] in the course of work on the general theory of drug action. He has found that many aspects of drug action are explained by the hypothesis that the magnitude of a stimulant action depends on the rate at which the drug makes contact with receptors. Earlier theories have supposed that the magnitude of the stimulant action depended on the total number of receptors occupied by molecules of the drug. But Paton has pointed out that if molecules of a drug remain in contact with receptors, by so doing they reduce the number of receptors which are free, and thus reduce the opportunities for stimulation. For a drug to be an effective stimulant, it must be able to dissociate itself from the receptors as quickly as possible after making contact with them. In this way the number of free receptors is kept high, and the rate at which the drug can

C

make contact with them is undiminished. In practice, however, the dissociation of the drug is never as fast as the process of association. The escape of the drug from the receptor is always slower than the approach to it. This is probably because the approach is determined simply by the attraction between the positively-charged $-\overset{+}{N}(CH_3)_3$ group and the negatively-charged receptor. But once contact has been made, escape is delayed by forces (van der Waals forces) exerted between the rest of the molecule and the receptor.

Thus, while the first application of a drug produces stimulation, later applications produce less and less stimulation because molecules of the drug remain attached to the receptors; if the rate of dissociation is low, the number of free receptors is continually reduced. Finally there is block.

When the drug makes contact with the receptor at first, it stimulates because of the depolarization which follows the contact. When this depolarization is prolonged, block of transmission may be due to the depolarization. However, when the contact between drug and receptor persists, there is no further depolarizing influence, and repolarization occurs. Transmission is, however, blocked by the persistent occupation of the receptors. This is often expressed by saying that a depolarizing block becomes a competitive block.

The substance tetramethylammonium differs from tetraethylammonium. The latter has a blocking action only, with no initial stimulant action [21]. For a stimulant action to be seen, at least two methyl groups must be attached to the quaternary nitrogen.

Ganglionic blocking agents. By far the most important development in the study of ganglionic transmission has been the discovery of agents which block transmission through the ganglion without causing depolarization, and which can be used in patients for this purpose. Tetraethylammonium was tested for its power to block transmission in patients but was found to be of little practical value. However, in 1948 Paton and Zaimis [22] found that hexamethonium was a far more useful substance.

After the isolation of d-tubocurarine in 1935 by King, a study of its structure showed that it contained two quaternary nitrogen atoms separated by ten other atoms; the molecule was, however, complex. Substances were then synthesized in which two methonium groups $-\overset{+}{N}(CH_3)_3$ were separated by a straight methylene chain, and these substances were tested for activity like that of d-tubocurarine at the neuromuscular junction. It was found indeed that when there were ten $-CH_2-$ groups in the chain the substance which was called decamethonium had a powerful blocking action at the neuromuscular junction. Paton and Zaimis then found that when there were six $-CH_2-$ groups in the chain the substance which was called hexamethonium had a powerful blocking action in the ganglion. Hexamethonium competes for the receptors on which acetylcholine acts, and acetylcholine, released from the terminations of the preganglionic fibres, is ineffective in stimulating the ganglion cells, which it can no longer depolarize. Thus hexamethonium blocks by competition, just as tetraethylammonium does.

Use of hexamethonium in hypertension. Hexamethonium was the first substance with which it was possible to control high blood pressure and to reverse the eye changes, the retinal haemorrhages and papilloedema formerly believed to be irreversible. It was usually given by mouth, but as it contains two quaternary nitrogen atoms, it was absorbed poorly from the gastro-intestinal tract, and patients needed progressively larger doses. It produced unpleasant symptoms by blocking parasympathetic ganglia as well as sympathetic ganglia, and patients constantly complained of dry mouth and of constipation. Often they suffered from disturbances of vision due to block of transmission through the ciliary ganglion. Later it was found that a better control of the blood pressure was obtained by intramuscular injection [23], when the doses were much less and could be kept at the same level for long periods though the side effects of dry mouth and blurred vision remained. After each injection there was a period of postural hypotension, which still remains a drawback of all more recently introduced agents, with the exception of α-methyldopa.

Postural hypotension is the fall of blood pressure which occurs when a patient under treatment with hexamethonium stands up. Ordinarily, on standing up, there is increased vasoconstriction in the splanchnic area resulting from a reflex initiated in the carotid sinus by the lowered pressure. When hexamethonium or other similar agent is effecting a block in ganglionic transmission, vasoconstriction in the splanchnic area cannot occur when the patient stands. As a result less blood goes to the head, the patient feels dizzy and may faint.

Accordingly, when patients with hypertension are treated with hexamethonium by intramuscular injection, they are warned to remain lying down for the first two or three hours, and to get up only when the effect of the drug is diminishing.

Other agents for producing ganglion block. Various other substances have been introduced and have been widely used as ganglion blocking agents; two which have proved better than hexamethonium because of greater potency are pentolinium and chlorisondamine.

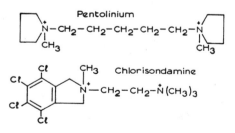

Both pentolinium and chlorisondamine contain two quaternary nitrogen atoms and therefore are at a disadvantage for oral administration, not being readily absorbed. However, an important step forward was made by the discovery that a substance which was a secondary amine, mecamylamine, had powerful activity as a ganglion-blocking agent. Mecamylamine is much more readily absorbed and therefore is effective by mouth in much lower dose than the quaternary nitrogen compounds. The greater ease of absorption, however, brought with it a new complication, because the change from a quaternary nitrogen compound to a secondary amine not only facilitated absorption from the gastro-intestinal tract, but facilitated entry into the brain. Mecamylamine in too large a dose produces tremor in patients because of a central action which hexamethonium and its successors do not possess. Pempidine is a second substance which does not contain quaternary nitrogen, and which is similar in action to mecamylamine, though pempidine has a shorter duration, which is sometimes an advantage.

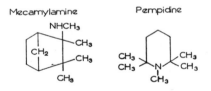

The duration of the action of mecamylamine and of pempidine is increased when they are given together with a diuretic which increases the alkalinity of the urine. Such a diuretic is chlorothiazide which increases the excretion of sodium by the kidney, and in doing so makes the urine more alkaline. The excretion of mecamylamine and of pempidine is then delayed. Substances related to chlorothiazide have a similar action.

Effect of adrenaline on ganglionic transmission. Adrenaline has two effects on ganglionic transmission. The first one to be observed was depression [199]. The second one to be observed was augmentation [200]. A beautiful paper by Bülbring [201] described both effects in the perfused superior cervical ganglion. De Groat and Volle [225] have shown that the depression produced by adrenaline is due to hyperpolarization of the ganglion, an effect which is blocked by alpha blocking agents. They also found that the augmentor effect facilitating ganglionic transmission was due to ganglionic depolarization by adrenaline, and that this action was blocked by beta-blocking agents.

CHAPTER 4

TRANSMISSION AT THE NEUROMUSCULAR JUNCTION

The liberation of acetylcholine. Although the events which occur at the neuromuscular junction in skeletal muscle are unconnected with the autonomic system, they were determined in close relation to the events in the autonomic system, and are therefore discussed briefly here. Great progress has been made in studying the details of transmission at the neuromuscular junction. The motor nerves terminate in small depressions on the muscle surface in which structures are present known as endplates. These are the parts of the muscle surface which are specifically sensitive to acetylcholine. In the nerve terminals beyond the end of the myelin sheath, a large number of vesicles have been seen by the aid of the electron microscope. From the work of Fatt and Katz [24] it appears that acetylcholine is being liberated not only when a nerve impulse arrives, but also during the intervening periods. A random succession of very small depolarizations is recorded at the endplate, each one identical in form with an endplate potential, and almost certainly due to acetylcholine perhaps released by the spontaneous disruption of a vesicle.

However, this release is very small compared to the release which follows the arrival of a nerve impulse. The acetylcholine released by the nerve impulse alters the endplate surface in such a way that it becomes freely permeable to the ions on each side of it. There is apparently some chemical breakdown of a local ion barrier which occurs as soon as acetylcholine combines with it. Thus acetylcholine short-circuits the endplate and thereby discharges the surrounding muscle membrane and gives rise to a propagated spike [118]. This spike, propagated over the muscle fibres, depends upon an increase in permeability which is specific for sodium. The contraction follows in its wake.

Substances which prevent the release of acetylcholine. The release of acetylcholine by stimulation of the motor nerve can be studied by using the diaphragm of the rat removed from the body together with the phrenic nerve [25]. When this preparation is set up in an isolated organ bath, the acetylcholine which is released on stimulation can be measured [119]. A substance which prevents the release is botulinum toxin. When this is added to the bath, the response to nerve stimulation gradually declines until it disappears. At this point the amount of acetylcholine released into the bath by a given stimulation is greatly reduced. Botulinum toxin does not affect conduction along the nerve and does not affect the muscle contraction; it therefore acts at the junction. However, it does not interfere with the synthesis of acetylcholine, nor does it interfere with the action of acetylcholine on the muscle. It thus seems to interfere with the release of acetylcholine.

Botulinum toxin owes its poisonous action in man to its effect in paralysing the terminations of cholinergic nerves.

A second substance which prevents the release of acetylcholine at the terminations of motor nerves is hemicholinium. The mechanism of its action has already been discussed. Its effect is to cause a decline in the response to nerve stimulation at a rate determined by the frequency of stimulation. When the frequency is low, the rate of decline is slow, and when the frequency is high, the rate of decline is rapid. Hemicholinium prevents the transport of choline to the site of synthesis of acetylcholine.

Triethylcholine. A recent observation [26] is that a much simpler substance than hemicholinium, namely triethylcholine, has the same effect. In choline three methyl groups are attached to the nitrogen atom; in triethylcholine, the methyl groups are replaced by ethyl groups. In the presence of triethylcholine, rapid stimulation of motor nerves to skeletal muscles leads to muscular weakness. A dog injected with triethylcholine can walk without any sign of difficulty, but soon after it begins to run it becomes so weak that it cannot stand. When triethylcholine is added to the bath containing a phrenic nerve-diaphragm preparation, the contractions induced by stimulation of the nerve decline in size, but can be restored by choline. It may be that choline acetylase makes the acetic ester of triethylcholine instead of the acetic ester of choline.

Cholinesterase. There are two enzymes which break down acetylcholine into choline and acetic acid, which were originally known as true and pseudo-cholinesterase. True cholinesterase is also called acetylcholinesterase and specific cholinesterase. It is present in the central nervous system in the supraoptic nucleus, in ganglia and in motor endplates. In these it is present in the synaptic gap and also in the postsynaptic membrane. Pseudo-cholinesterase is also called non-specific and butyrylcholinesterase. It is present in plasma, in the intestinal mucosa and also in the central nervous system.

The action of eserine. Eserine inhibits the action of cholinesterase by combining with it. However, the inhibition does not last long, since the cholinesterase destroys the eserine. Thus eserine competes with acetylcholine for the enzyme. The effect of inhibiting the cholinesterase is to convert the response of the muscle to a single nerve impulse into a repetitive discharge. In the phrenic nerve-diaphragm two effects of eserine are seen. When the nerve is stimulated at a slow rate of 5 per min. the contractions increase in size when eserine is added to the bath. The increase is due to a change from a single twitch in response to a single nerve volley to a tetanus in response to a repetitive volley. If, however, the rate of stimulation is increased to 50 per minute while eserine is still present, the contractions then steadily decline. This decline occurs because at the high frequency the acetylcholine accumulates in the presence of eserine and causes a block of neuromuscular transmission due to a steady diminution of the number of free receptors.

Eserine is mainly used in clinical work to treat glaucoma. In this condition sight is endangered by a rise in pressure in the anterior chamber of the eye. When eserine (physostigmine) is put in the conjunctival sac, it is absorbed and diminishes the rate at which acetylcholine, released at the terminations of the IIIrd nerve, is destroyed. As a result the sphincter of the iris contracts more than before. This causes a widening of the Canal of Schlemm and allows increased drainage from the anterior chamber of the eye. The ciliary muscle also contracts and therefore the suspensory ligament relaxes. The lens becomes more spherical, and distant vision is blurred.

The action of neostigmine. Neostigmine is commonly classed with eserine, but its action is of longer duration and is more complicated. In clinical work it is of much greater use. Not only does it potentiate the action of acetylcholine by inhibiting cholinesterase, but it also acts on the presynaptic segment of the neuromuscular junction. Neostigmine facilitates a repetitive response in the presynaptic segment, which is the termination of the motor nerve not surrounded by a myelin sheath. An important study has been made by Riker [27].

Neostigmine has two main uses in clinical work, first to increase muscular strength in myasthenia gravis, and second to neutralize the action of tubocurarine or gallamine at the end of a surgical operation when the patient does not breathe spontaneously, or when his breathing is inadequate. For these latter purposes, the injection of neostigmine must always be preceded

by the injection of atropine to exclude the effects of acetylcholine which accumulates at the parasympathetic endings.
Otherwise neostigmine will slow the heart and diminish the
blood pressure. Atropine takes some time to act, though the
delay is reduced when it is given intravenously. Moreover, it is
commonly given in too small a dose such as 0·6 mg. A dose
which is fully effective in man is 2 mg.

Edrophonium is a substance having an action like that of
neostigmine. Its formula is

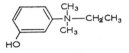

Edrophonium is useful in the diagnosis of myasthenia gravis;
when injected into such a patient, it quickly increases the power
of the muscles; this is noticed first in the eyelids which no longer
remain half closed. The action of edrophonium is of much
shorter duration than that of neostigmine.

War gases. A series of substances with powerful anticholinesterase action have been synthesized chiefly for use in chemical
warfare. They are also important as insecticides. One of the
best known of these is di-isopropylfluorophosphonate (dyflos):

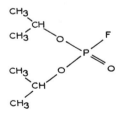

This substance has the peculiarity that when it is injected
intravenously it does not become distributed throughout the

body, but is attached to the first tissues which it meets. It is thus of no use in the treatment of myasthenia gravis. However, when an intra-arterial injection of dyflos is given to a patient with myasthenia gravis, the muscles supplied by the artery, but not others, recover full power and retain it for perhaps three weeks. Its combination with cholinesterase is very firm and it was believed to be irreversible, but now drugs are known which protect against poisoning. The best is pyridine 2-aldoxime.

The action of tubocurarine. It has been known since the experiments of Claude Bernard, made over one hundred years ago, that the S. American arrow poison curare was able to block the neuromuscular junction. The substance tubocurarine was isolated as a pure substance in 1935. It produces a block without causing depolarization, by competing with acetylcholine for the receptors in the postsynaptic membrane. Tubocurarine affects muscles in a regular order. The muscles of the eyelids and the small muscles of the hand are affected first, then the large limb muscles; third the intercostal muscles and fourth the diaphragm. Tubocurarine contains two quaternary nitrogen atoms at a distance of $14\overset{\circ}{\mathrm{A}}$.

Action of succinylcholine. Decamethonium contains two methonium, $-\overset{+}{\mathrm{N}}(CH_3)_3$, groups joined by a chain of ten $-CH_2-$ groups. This substance causes neuromuscular block in the first place by causing depolarization, but later maintains the block in some other way; a reduction in the excitability of the muscle near the endplates has been suggested. Decamethonium is not used very much, but the substance succinylcholine, which has a similar action, is used a great deal in anaesthesia.

$$(CH_3)_3\overset{+}{\mathrm{N}}-CH_2-CH_2-O-CO-CH_2-CH_2-CO-O-CH_2-CH_2\overset{+}{\mathrm{N}}(CH_3)_3$$

This substance is hydrolyzed by pseudocholinesterase and therefore its action is of short duration. It is useful to anaesthetists because when it is injected it enables an endotracheal tube to be passed into position without difficulty, and its action soon comes to an end. However, there are patients in whom the action lasts for a long time. It is commonly believed that these are deficient in plasma cholinesterase, and cannot hydrolyze the succinylcholine. Decamethonium causes muscle fasciculation, though it is transient.

Action of gallamine. A synthetic curarizing agent with an action like that of tubocurarine is gallamine. It does not cause depolarization and does not cause fasciculation. Its formula is

It causes some acceleration of the heart, which may be due to block of vagal ganglia. Tubocurarine occasionally has some ganglion-blocking action, seen as a fall of blood pressure; tubocurarine may also cause a fall of blood pressure by release of histamine. In spite of the effect on the heart, which is not severe, gallamine is much used as a long-acting muscle relaxant.

Effect of anaesthetics and of temperature on blocking agents. The relation of the volatile anaesthetics to the action of muscle relaxants is important. Ether, by its own action, reduces the contractions of skeletal muscle, whether the nerve is given single shocks or tetanic stimulation. Tubocurarine has a greater depressant action on the neuromuscular junction in the presence of ether. Cyclopropane and halothane do not themselves depress muscle contractions, but in their presence tubocurarine has a greater action [120].

The effect of temperature depends on the drugs which are used. The effect of the drugs which are said to block by competition, namely tubocurarine and gallamine, is less at a lower temperature. On the other hand the effect of depolarizing drugs like succinylcholine (suxamethonium) is greater at a lower temperature. These statements refer to man [121].

The action of adrenaline. Adrenaline has long been known to affect transmission at the neuromuscular junction. Orbeli and Ginetinsky showed that repeated stimulation of the motor roots led to a diminishing response. When the sympathetic fibres were stimulated in addition, the response recovered. Later it was shown that adrenaline had the same effect. When a motor nerve is stimulated for a prolonged period, a failure of conduction occurs which is intermittent, and which is located in the presynaptic terminals [28]. For example, not more than 60 per cent of the impulses may be transmitted. However, when adrenaline is given the percentage of impulses which are transmitted rises to 100. Adrenaline restores presynaptic conduction even when the muscle contractions are abolished by tubocurarine.

Adrenaline causes the release of an increased amount of acetylcholine. Its effect is readily demonstrated in an anaesthetized cat when the sciatic nerve is stimulated at a rate of 6 shocks per minute and the increase of tension in the gastrocnemius muscle is recorded. After the injection of 10 μg. neostigmine (which by itself is without effect) the injection of 40 μg. adrenaline then causes a rise in the tension which may be as much as 0·5 kg. [202]. Recently it has been shown that the combined effect of adrenaline and neostigmine in increasing muscle tension is greatly increased by theophylline. This indicates that the effect of adrenaline is likely to be exerted through the formation of cyclic AMP (see page 49). (See also Bowman and Raper [203] for an effect of adrenaline on curarized muscle stimulated directly.)

Various observers have stated that the treatment of myasthenia gravis by neostigmine is improved by giving ephedrine in addition. Since ephedrine liberates noradrenaline, the benefit following the administration of ephedrine may be due to the action of noradrenaline in improving presynaptic conduction.

CHAPTER 5

THE FORMATION OF ADRENALINE

The work of Cannon. The discovery that the adrenal medulla contained a substance which was very active in raising the blood pressure was made by Oliver and Schäfer in 1894. It is interesting to observe that the discovery was made independently by two other physiologists in other places within a few months. These were Szymonowicz and Cybulski. The time was evidently ripe for the discovery to be made.

In the year in which Loewi demonstrated the liberation of 'accelerans-stoff' when he stimulated the vago-sympathetic trunk running to the atropinized heart of the toad, Cannon and Uridil were demonstrating a similar effect by a different method. They were engaged in replying to the statements of two other American physiologists, Stewart and Rogoff, who did not believe that stimulation of the splanchnic nerves liberated adrenaline from the adrenal medulla. Cannon used as an index of the liberation of adrenaline the rate of the cat heart, which had been denervated at an earlier operation. In such a cat the heart rate could increase only as a result of the action of a substance carried in the blood. Cannon and Uridil found that when the splanchnic nerves were stimulated in a large number of cats, the heart rate rose by a mean figure of 29 beats per minute. They removed the adrenal glands, and then found that the heart rate rose by a mean figure of only 6 beats per minute [29].

Cannon was curious to know why there was any rise at all. He wondered what the substance was which then entered the blood to cause the small rise of 6 beats per minute. He showed

39

that the rise occurred after clamping the aorta and the vena cava just above the renal arteries, provided that the nerves to the liver were intact. He concluded that the substance was liberated from the endings of nerves running to the liver. That was in 1921. Nine years later Cannon and Bacq [30] demonstrated by somewhat elaborate but very clear experiments that when the sympathetic fibres to the tail of the cat were stimulated, a rise in the rate of the denervated heart occurred. They showed that a substance was liberated from the sympathetic terminations in the tail which was carried in the blood to the heart, and caused the rate to rise. They called the substance Sympathin. Later Cannon and Rosenblueth came to the conclusion that Sympathin was not one, but two substances, one having motor effects and the other inhibitory effects. Subsequent work showed, however, that there was in the main only one substance.

The work of Euler. While it was agreed that Sympathin must be chemically similar to adrenaline, the evidence which was available showed that it was not adrenaline. In 1946 U. S. von Euler [31] extracted the splenic nerves of the ox and of the horse and showed that the extract behaved like a solution of noradrenaline, which lacks the methyl group attached to the nitrogen atom in adrenaline, but is otherwise the same. Euler's view that noradrenaline was the substance which was liberated from sympathetic nerve endings was confirmed by the demonstration that stimulation of the splenic nerves liberated noradrenaline [32].

Noradrenaline was also found to be present in the adrenal medulla. When an extract of the adrenal medulla was matched with adrenaline on the blood pressure of the cat, 1 ml. of the extract being equivalent to a certain amount of adrenaline, it was found that this relation did not hold when tests were made on the blood sugar. The adrenaline had more effect in raising the blood sugar. This was explained by the presence of much noradrenaline in the extract, which was powerful in raising the blood pressure, but weak in raising the blood sugar [33].

The formation of noradrenaline and adrenaline. The steps leading to the formation of adrenaline were forecast independently by Blaschko [204] and by Holtz [205]. The first evidence was obtained by Demis, Blaschko and Welch [206]. The steps are shown in Table 5.1. The amino-acid phenylalanine is converted to tyrosine by hydroxylation in the ring. Tyrosine is converted to dihydroxyphenylalanine (called dopa for short) by a second hydroxylation in the ring. The hydroxyl groups are then in the 3 and 4 positions. Dopa is decarboxylated, and

TABLE 5.1.

Formation of adrenaline

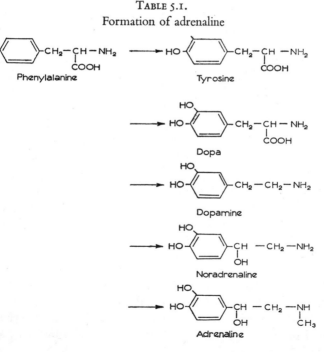

becomes the amine dihydroxyphenylethylamine, or dopamine. Finally dopamine is again hydroxylated, an –OH group being attached to the carbon atom in the side-chain which is next to the ring. The result is noradrenaline. When a methyl group is substituted in the –NH₂ group, noradrenaline becomes adrenaline.

The first step, in which phenylalanine is converted to tyrosine, offers difficulty in some persons, due to an inborn metabolic error, a single enzyme being lacking, and tyrosine cannot be produced. The phenylalanine is then converted to phenylpyruvic acid and phenylacetic acid, and these are excreted in the urine. The condition in which this happens is called **phenylketonuria.** Now tyrosine is not only the first step in the formation of noradrenaline and adrenaline, but it is also the starting point of the formation of the pigment melanin. The result is that patients suffering from phenylketonuria are deficient in noradrenaline and adrenaline, and are also unpigmented. Tyrosine is also a starting point in the formation of the thyroid hormone, so that the hormone is lacking. In addition there is a defect in the formation of 5-hydroxytryptamine. Perhaps the deficient enzyme normally converts tryptophan to 5-hydroxytryptophan. Children with phenylketonuria are backward in their mental development. This may be due to lack of thyroid hormone, or, as some think, to lack of 5-hydroxytryptamine.

The tyrosine–dopa conversion. The step which limits the rate of noradrenaline synthesis is the conversion of tyrosine to dopa. This is effected by an enzyme called **tyrosine hydroxylase** [149]. It was found that the conversion of tyrosine to dopa was inhibited by α-methyl tyrosine, and when this substance was given to guinea-pigs, the amount of dopamine and of noradrenaline in the brain stem, in the caudate nucleus, in the heart and in the spleen could be reduced to undetectable levels. In such animals neither tyramine nor noradrenaline caused a rise of blood pressure. Tyramine acts by releasing noradrenaline, and when there was none to release, tyramine was inactive. Noradrenaline is taken up by sympathetic postganglionic fibres, and when these were empty, noradrenaline was taken up so avidly that it was unable to cause a rise of pressure (see p. 57). Tyrosine hydroxylase inhibitors are used in the treatment of adrenal medullary tumours (phaeochromocytoma) to deplete them of catecholamines.

The dopa-dopamine conversion. An important step is the conversion of the amino-acid dihydroxyphenylalanine, commonly known as dopa, into the amine known as dopamine. This change converts a substance which is without pharmacological activity into one which is pharmacologically active. Thus dopa has no action on the blood pressure, while dopamine has a weak action on the blood pressure.

Dopamine on the blood pressure. The actual direction in which dopamine changes the blood pressure depends on the circumstances in which it is tested. In the cat under ether with the vagi cut, when the blood pressure is high, dopamine causes a fall of blood pressure. In the rabbit or guinea-pig under urethane, dopamine also causes a fall of blood pressure. However, in a spinal cat, when the blood pressure is low, dopamine causes a rise of blood pressure. The difference in the action depends on the extent to which the blood vessels are under the influence of noradrenaline when dopamine arrives. Noradrenaline can be removed from the blood vessels by treating the animal with reserpine (see p. 53). The injection of dopamine into a cat under ether with the vagi cut, no longer causes a fall of blood pressure if the cat has previously been treated with reserpine. It causes a rise. Similarly the injection of dopamine into a rabbit or guinea-pig under urethane causes a rise of blood pressure if the animal has been treated beforehand with reserpine. Thus when the receptors in the blood vessels' walls are not occupied with noradrenaline, dopamine acts on the receptors and causes

43

a rise of pressure. However, when the receptors are already occupied with noradrenaline, and the vessels are contracted under its influence, the arrival of dopamine displaces some of the noradrenaline. Since the activity of dopamine in causing constriction is less than that of noradrenaline, the displacement of the noradrenaline by dopamine results in a relaxation of the vascular tone.

Hence dopamine may cause a rise of blood pressure or a fall, depending on the circumstances [122]. The term 'partial agonist' has been applied to substances which act in this way. Two substances may have the same 'affinity' for receptors, and yet one of them when combined with the receptors has a greater 'efficacy' than the other in causing contraction [123].

In Parkinson's disease (see p. 86) L-dopa is administered to patients in order to increase dopamine in the corpus striatum. The L-dopa is given by mouth, and produces much dopamine outside as well as inside the brain. It is common to observe a lowering of blood pressure in these patients.

The action of α-methyl dopa. The conversion of dopa into dopamine is also the conversion of a substance which easily enters the brain (by passing the so-called blood-brain barrier) into one which enters the brain with much more difficulty. Amines like dopamine, noradrenaline and adrenaline do not readily enter the brain.

The conversion of dopa into dopamine is effected by an enzyme which brings about decarboxylation of dopa; the enzyme is dopa decarboxylase. Now the carbon atom in dopa to which the –COOH group is attached is known as the α carbon. If a –CH$_3$ group is substituted for the hydrogen on the α carbon, the substance α-methyl dopa is obtained.

Alpha-methyl dopa was found to inhibit the decarboxylation of dopa and to have sedative properties in man. It lowered the blood pressure. Moreover it inhibited the synthesis of serotonin

(5HT) in patients with carcinoid tumours. In the body it appears to be converted to α-methyl dopamine, and this in its turn is converted into α-methyl noradrenaline. Thus when α-methyl dopa is given to patients, the normal conversion of dopa to noradrenaline occurs side by side with a conversion of α-methyl dopa to α-methyl noradrenaline. Both the noradrenaline and the α-methyl noradrenaline are taken up by the sympathetic nerve endings, and when sympathetic impulses arrive both substances are released. However, α-methyl noradrenaline is less active than noradrenaline (on some organs much less active) and therefore the effect of a given stimulation is less [124].

The properties of the catechol amines. There are four important catechol amines, of which three are present in the body. These are dopamine, noradrenaline and adrenaline. The fourth is a product of the laboratory. To the nitrogen atom of noradrenaline an isopropyl group is attached. Since noradrenaline is also called arterenol in the United States, this substance is N-isopropyl arterenol; this name has been shortened to isoproterenol. In Britain it is called isoprenaline, which is a shortened form of isopropyl noradrenaline.

The following are different names for these catechol amines:

1. Dihydroxyphenylethylamine.
   Dopamine.
   Hydroxytyramine.
   (Epinine is N-methyl dopamine.)

2. Dihydroxyphenylethanolamine.
   Noradrenaline.
   Norepinephrine.
   Arterenol.
   (Levarterenol is the naturally occurring laevo form.)

3. N-methyl dihydroxyphenylethanolamine.
   Adrenaline.
   Epinephrine.

4. N-isopropyl noradrenaline.
   Isoprenaline.
   N-isopropylarterenol.
   Isoproterenol.

Dopamine is an amine with much less physiological activity than noradrenaline. The insertion of an –OH group on the carbon atom next to the ring in dopamine causes a great increase in physiological activity, from 50 to 150 times according to the conditions in which the comparison is made. Dopamine is present in the corpus striatum except in Parkinsonism, when it is absent, although the anatomical structure is unchanged (see Chapter 9). Patients then have involuntary movements and other motor disabilities such as akinesia, when an effort to move has a slow beginning.

It is not known how disturbances of dopamine metabolism interfere with normal motility, but *normal motor function depends on normal function of neurones producing dopamine.*

Noradrenaline, Adrenaline and Isoprenaline. The catechol amines noradrenaline, adrenaline and isoprenaline differ in their properties. In a general way it can be said that in smooth muscle noradrenaline has motor properties, that adrenaline has both motor and inhibitor properties, while isoprenaline has only inhibitor properties. For example, in the treatment of asthma a substance is required which will relax the muscles of the bronchioles. Noradrenaline is not used, because its relaxing or inhibitor action on bronchial musculature is too weak. Adrenaline is about forty times stronger than noradrenaline in causing bronchial inhibition, and therefore adrenaline is used. Isoprenaline is about nine times stronger than adrenaline, and so is the best of the three substances; it is, of course, also used.

An even more striking gradation of properties is seen when the blood pressure is considered. In the cat anaesthetized with ether, when the vagi are cut, the blood pressure is high. An injection of a small dose of noradrenaline causes a rise of blood pressure above the already high level. An injection of a small dose of adrenaline, however, causes a fall. An injection of isoprenaline also causes a fall. In a spinal cat, in which the brain has been destroyed, the blood pressure is maintained at a rather low level so long as artificial respiration is given. In a spinal cat, noradrenaline and also adrenaline cause a rise of blood pressure, but isoprenaline causes a fall.

CHAPTER 6

THE ACTION OF ADRENALINE

The action of cyclic AMP. The discovery of cyclic AMP, which has explained many of the actions of adrenaline, began with the interest of E. W. Sutherland in the increase in blood sugar which follows the injection of adrenaline. It was first found that the level of hexose phosphates increased in liver slices when either adrenaline or glucagon was added. The conclusion was drawn that glucose was derived from glycogen and that the enzyme phosphorylase was activated in response to adrenaline or glucagon. In broken cell preparations they were at first unable to demonstrate the process of activation, but they succeeded in demonstrating the opposite process of inactivation of active phosphorylase, and they were able to purify an enzyme, a phosphatase, which did this.

Thus it appeared that the action of adrenaline and glucagon in activating phosphorylase might involve phosphorylation of inactive enzymes, and this was demonstrated in liver slices. Later, by adding ATP and magnesium ions, they were able to demonstrate this effect of the hormones in broken cell preparations. Thus the state of liver phosphorylase represented a balance between a kinase, which activated the enzyme, and a phosphatase, which inactivated it.

When the material was centrifuged and the precipitate was removed, adrenaline and glucagon did not cause the activation. Instead they reacted with some component of the precipitate to stimulate the production of a heat-stable factor found to be adenosine $3',5'$ monophosphate or cyclic AMP.

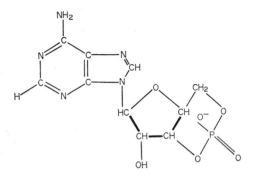

Formula of cyclic AMP

The relation of adrenaline to ATP was established by Sutherland and Rall [209] and Sutherland and Robinson [210] who showed that adrenaline stimulates the enzyme adenyl cyclase to transform ATP to cyclic AMP.

Cyclic AMP is destroyed by a phosphodiesterase which converts the cyclic compound to inactive 5-AMP. The action of the phosphodiesterase is inhibited by caffeine and theophylline, so that in the presence of either of these substances the effect of cyclic AMP is greatly increased.

Further actions of cyclic AMP. The addition of cyclic AMP to liver slices had the same effect as adrenaline and glucagon in stimulating the release of glucose, and Haynes showed that ACTH, but not of course adrenaline or glucagon, stimulated the formation of cyclic AMP in the adrenal cortex; he further showed that cyclic AMP could stimulate steroid formation when applied to adrenal cortical slices.

The hormones known or thought to produce some of their effects through cyclic AMP also include vasopressin, thyrotrophin, luteinizing hormone, melanocyte-stimulating hormone and parathyroid hormone. The hormones themselves are the first messenger, and travel to the target cells where they interact with specific receptors, some closely related to adenyl cyclase. Cyclic AMP is then formed and this serves as a second messenger. It is suggested that all of the diverse effects of this nucleotide are due to its ability to increase the activity of intracellular protein kinases.

Other actions of adrenaline. Not only does adrenaline liberate glucose from the liver through the action of cyclic AMP, but it increases the intracellular concentration of cyclic AMP at the same time as it increases the contractile force of the heart, and as it increases the release of fatty acid from adipose tissue. Effects of adrenaline within the nervous system may also be mediated by cyclic AMP. Thus adrenaline enhances transmission of impulses passing down the sciatic nerve to the gastrocnemius in the cat. This is best seen in the presence of an anticholinesterase. This effect of adrenaline is potentiated by theophylline, sometimes as much as tenfold. The potentiation is blocked by propranolol and does not occur in the curarized preparation [215].

The action of imidazole. Butcher and Sutherland have shown that imidazole (0·05 M) activates the phosphodiesterase which causes hydrolysis of cyclic AMP. In the presence of imidazole adrenaline fails to produce its physiological effect on the taenia, and it also fails to increase the ATP and creatine phosphate content of the tissue. The action of adrenaline is not abolished by histamine concentrations which produce a similar rise in tone as imidazole. [Bueding and Bülbring, 208.]

The double effect of adrenaline. Adrenaline causes some forms of smooth muscle to contract and others to relax. Thus it causes contraction of the uterus of the non-pregnant rabbit, but relaxes the uterus of the non-pregnant cat. If the transmembrane potential across the cell membrane of skeletal muscle fibres is measured it is usually 90 mV, at which figure it remains steady until an impulse arrives which causes depolarization. Until an impulse arrives the muscle is relaxed, the membrane being almost impermeable to sodium. The transmembrane potential is mainly the result of the difference between the high potassium concentration inside and the low potassium concentration outside. Much work on smooth muscle has been done on the taenia coli, which is a strip of muscle running along the caecum of the guinea-pig. The fibres are parallel to one another. In this muscle the transmembrane potential changes continually, rising and falling around an average figure of about 50 mV. This value varies according to the muscle and its condition. Thus in the uterus of the ovariectomized rat it is 35 mV, while in the uterus of the rat in oestrus it is 57 mV. These figures, which are so much lower than the figure for skeletal muscle, are partly due to a lower permeability of the cell membrane to potassium, and partly to a higher permeability for sodium.

The transmembrane potential, being already low, is unstable and when it falls it often reaches the threshold level at which an action potential or spike is discharged. This occurs spontaneously and is not due to propagation of impulses from an endplate as in skeletal muscle. These spontaneous action potentials are conducted from cell to cell. A spike initiates a contraction, and the tension developed depends on the frequency at which the spikes occur. When a series of spikes has occurred, they stop, the transmembrane potential rises and the muscle relaxes. Thus the alternation of a falling transmembrane potential with a series of spikes, and of a rising transmembrane potential with no spikes, is responsible for the continual rise and fall in tension which is characteristic of smooth muscle. This rise and fall in the transmembrane potential appears to be due to the relative inefficiency of active processes at the membrane which stabilize the transmembrane potential. There is not sufficient energy available to keep the muscle relaxed.

Adrenaline and energy supply. Adrenaline, when applied to the taenia, causes a rise in the transmembrane potential, a cessation of action potentials (that is of 'spikes') and a relaxation of muscle tension. Bülbring [207] suggested that these changes might be brought about by an increased supply and utilization of metabolic energy. She pointed out that there was a striking similarity between the effect of adrenaline and the effect of a sudden rise of temperature, and also the effect of the addition of glucose after a period of glucose deficiency. Both these changes caused a cessation of spontaneous contractions, a rise in the transmembrane potential, and made the membrane inexcitable and more stable. The opposite effects were produced by sudden cooling, by removing glucose, by metabolic inhibitors such as mono-iodoacetate, and by strophanthin which inhibits the sodium pump.

In other smooth muscles, as for example in the non-pregnant uterus of the rabbit, in the nictitating membrane of the cat or in the bladder of the ferret, adrenaline has another effect, which is due to depolarization, causing contraction. This depolarizing effect is usually seen when the transmembrane potential is high, while on the other hand the hyperpolarizing effect, which causes relaxation, is seen when the transmembrane potential is low.

The two actions of adrenaline can be seen in the same tissue, for example in the smooth muscle of the arteries of the cat. In a cat under ether anaesthesia, when the vagi are cut, the blood pressure is usually high, perhaps exceeding 200 mm. of mercury. Small doses of adrenaline, e.g. 2·5 μg. or 5 μg. then cause a fall of blood pressure presumably due to the increase in the transmembrane potential. In a cat in which the spinal cord has been divided at the 2nd cervical vertebra, and in which the brain has been destroyed, respiration being maintained artificially, doses of 10 μg. or 20 μg. adrenaline cause a rise in blood pressure, which is then about 100 mm. of mercury or less. This is the depolarizing action.

The blocking agents

Adrenaline reversal. Dale [218] discovered that in ergot there was an active principle which was capable of reversing the action of adrenaline on the blood pressure of the spinal cat. The effect of an intravenous injection of 20 μg. of adrenaline in such a cat was to cause an abrupt rise of blood pressure. When 0·5 mg. of the active principle (which was isolated by Barger and Carr as ergotoxine) was injected, and then, a few minutes later, the dose of adrenaline was repeated, it produced a very small rise. If then, at the top of this rise another injection of adrenaline was given, the blood pressure fell. Provided a sufficient amount of ergotoxine, which might sometimes be as much as 10 mg., was injected, even large doses of adrenaline caused only a fall of pressure. The effect of adrenaline on the blood pressure was completely reversed. (It may be noted that Stoll in 1921 isolated ergotamine, which had the same properties as ergotoxine; he stated that ergotoxine was a mixture of three substances, ergocornine, ergocristine and ergocryptine.)

Dale observed that although the constrictor action of adrenaline on the blood vessels had been abolished by ergotoxine, the accelerating action of adrenaline on the heart still remained; thus he found that there were some sites where ergotoxine abolished the action of adrenaline, and other sites where it did not affect the action. So far as smooth muscle was concerned the sites where ergotoxine had no effect were sites where adrenaline exerted an inhibitory action such as on the non-pregnant cat uterus. Sites where ergotoxine abolished or reversed the action of adrenaline were sites where adrenaline normally was motor.

Subsequently several other substances were found to have similar properties to ergotoxine or ergotamine; these included yohimbine, piperoxane, phentolamine, phenoxybenzamine and Hydergine (a proprietary compound which may be described as dihydro-ergotoxine).

Ahlquist's conception of alpha and beta receptors. After isoprenaline (isoproterenol) was introduced, Ahlquist [142] proposed that there were two kinds of receptors, alpha receptors on which adrenaline acted in causing motor effects which were blocked by ergotamine, and beta receptors on which adrenaline acted in producing inhibitory effects and effects on the heart which were not blocked by ergotamine. Substances like ergotamine, yohimbine, piperoxane, phenoxybenzamine and the others, soon became known as alpha blocking agents.

In 1958 Powell and Slater [219] introduced dichloroisoproterenol (DCI) as an antagonist of the inhibitory effects of adrenaline; this substance was soon found to antagonize the effects of adrenaline on cardiac rate and force. Thus DCI became the first beta blocking agent, to which others were added, for example pronethalol and more recently propranolol. The beta blocking agents mostly have the isoprenaline (isoproterenol) side chain, whereas the alpha blocking agents have no chemical structure in common.

Pronethalol was shown to have a very interesting property. When the cardiac glycoside ouabain is slowly infused into the vein of a guinea-pig, after a time the heart becomes rapid and very irregular, finally passing into ventricular fibrillation. However, when pronethalol was given beforehand, the occurrence of ventricular fibrillation was completely prevented [143]. This substance is not used because it was found to produce lymphosarcomas in mice.

The third substance is *propranolol* and has the formula

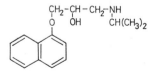

It is ten times more potent than pronethalol. It blocks the effect of isoprenaline in increasing the tension of the left ventricular

54

muscle in dogs. Further it antagonizes the increase in the rate of the sinoatrial node of the guinea-pig which is caused by adrenaline.

The clinical uses of propranolol are important. It is of great value in arresting paroxysmal tachycardia when the heart has recurrent periods of beating at a very high rate for some hours. It is of value in arresting cardiac irregularity during anaesthesia, and has been used successfully to stop ventricular fibrillation. There has been discussion whether this property is due to its beta-blocking action or whether it is due to its local anaesthetic property. Local anaesthetics, especially lignocaine, are used to suppress cardiac irregularities. Propranolol has been shown to benefit patients with angina pectoris who feel cardiac pain on exertion. When injected intravenously it was found to improve the exercise tolerance of these patients as measured by work on a bicycle ergometer. The heart rate was reduced at all levels of exercise, though the cardiac output in the erect position was maintained. Propranolol was also beneficial to those with angina when given by mouth for 2 weeks [151].

Propranolol has also been shown to reduce blood pressure in patients with hypertension, and was believed to have this effect because it prevented the sympathetic (cardiac) nerves from working. Thus it diminished the rate and force of the heart beats. An effective reduction of blood pressure was obtained in 15 out of 16 patients by giving doses from 100 to 400 mg. per day by mouth. There was no postural hypotension [152].

In many respects Ahlquist's definition has proved very useful. When the three substances noradrenaline, adrenaline and iso-prenaline are compared for their effects on the blood pressure, noradrenaline may be said to act mostly on alpha receptors and little on beta receptors, while adrenaline acts about equally on both. Thus in the presence of ergotamine the action of nor-adrenaline is greatly reduced, but not reversed, while the effect of adrenaline is reversed. Isoprenaline acts almost entirely on beta receptors causing a fall of blood pressure and is unaffected by ergotamine. Again on the bronchioles noradrenaline has very little dilator effect, and is of no use in the treatment of asthma; adrenaline has a good dilator action, and isoprenaline has an excellent dilator action.

The use to which the energy is put. In what way does the energy which is provided by the action of adrenaline lead to relaxation? There is evidence for the view that when Ca^{++} is absorbed on the membrane *effectively*, the membrane becomes less permeable to Na^+. Thus excess Ca^{++} increases the trans-membrane potential by reducing the permeability of the membrane to Na^+. A reduction of the external Na^+, or the addition of adrenaline to the solution, affects the transmembrane potential in the same way as excess of Ca^{++}. Thus it seems that the increased energy supplied by adrenaline may be used to improve the function of Ca^{++} at the membrane. By supplying energy, the Ca^{++} is held at the membrane, and the permeability of the membrane to Na^+ is diminished. The spike discharge ceases and the threshold for excitation rises. The result is hyperpolarization. In addition, adrenaline has been shown to increase the permeability of the cell membrane to potassium. However, the hyperpolarization which is observed under normal conditions opposes the outward movement of potassium. Therefore an increased efflux of potassium is rarely seen [216]. On the other hand, when the muscle is depolarized, the increased efflux of potassium in the presence of adrenaline is consistently observed [217]. Adrenaline thus causes relaxation of intestinal smooth muscle, partly as an effect on potassium permeability and partly as an effect which is secondary to the increase in metabolic energy which it produces.

Recently Jenkinson and Morton [217] have described results in which they have very successfully distinguished between the actions of noradrenaline and isoprenaline and also between the alpha blocker phentolamine and the beta blocker pronethalol in an unusual situation, namely at the smooth muscle membrane. They first studied the effect of noradrenaline and of isoprenaline on the rate of loss of ^{42}K from isolated strips of guinea-pig taenia, but found that their results were complicated by the hyperpolarizing action of the two substances. They therefore studied the loss of ^{42}K from strips which were depolarized by the presence of a high K^+ concentration (235 mM), and found that whereas noradrenaline greatly increased the rate of loss of ^{42}K, isoprenaline had no effect. This increase therefore appeared to be due to an effect on alpha receptors. The increased rate of loss was interpreted as an increase in the permeability of the cell membrane to K^+. The authors then made a different comparison. This was of the comparative effectiveness of noradrenaline and isoprenaline in inhibiting the contractures of taenia muscle which follow the addition of Ca^{++} to Ca^{++}-free K^+-rich bathing fluid. In this comparison isoprenaline was at least 30 times more active than noradrenaline. Thus the inhibition evidently involved the beta receptors rather than the alpha receptors.

These conclusions were confirmed by the use of blocking drugs. The effect of noradrenaline in inhibiting Ca^{++} contractures of depolarized taenia was strongly antagonized by the beta blocker pronethalol, but not at all by the alpha blocker phentolamine. However, when these same blocking agents were tested for their ability to antagonize the effect of noradrenaline on the efflux of $^{42}K^+$ through the cell membrane, phentolamine blocked the action of noradrenaline, but pronethalol had no effect. Thus the hypothesis that this action involved the alpha rather than the beta receptors was confirmed. The results of this research were clear and unambiguous, and afford an excellent example of the difference between alpha and beta receptors.

Adenyl cyclase as the beta receptor. The work of Jenkinson and Morton just described is however only one side of the picture, and other observations indicate that the alpha and beta receptors are much less distinct. Robison, Butcher and Sutherland [214] have pointed out that the properties of an alpha or beta receptor in one tissue are rarely if ever the same as the properties of a similar receptor in another tissue. (1) There is a variation from one species to another. Stimulation of glycogen breakdown in the liver is mediated by beta receptors in the dog, but by alpha receptors in the rat and rabbit. (2) Beta receptors leading to increased force of contraction in the heart are much more stimulated by noradrenaline than those leading to inhibition of mobility in the cat uterus. The uterine receptors are blocked by isopropylmethoxamine, but this substance is a very weak antagonist in the heart. (3) In smooth muscle stimulation of alpha receptors generally causes contraction, and stimulation of beta receptors causes inhibition. However, in the intestine stimulation of either leads to inhibition. (4) In the non-pregnant cat adrenaline causes relaxation, but if the cat is treated with progesterone, the beta receptors are overcome by alpha receptors, and adrenaline causes contraction.

Robison, Butcher and Sutherland [214] consider that it is at least possible that both alpha receptors and beta receptors may in reality be parts of an adenyl cyclase system. They suggest that 'perhaps the two types of receptors represent only the extremes of a continuum, near the centre of which stands the relatively indiscriminate adenylcyclase of adipose tissue'.

CHAPTER 7

THE FATE OF CATECHOL AMINES.
UPTAKE.
SUBSTANCES WHICH RELEASE
NORADRENALINE

The action of reserpine. Until a few years ago, the fate of noradrenaline and of adrenaline in the body was not known. The enzyme monoamine oxidase is present within the cells of many tissues, and some believed that this enzyme was responsible for inactivating the amines by splitting the amine group from the side chain

$$-CH_2 \cdot NH_2 + O = -CHO + NH_3$$

However, the rate of disappearance of noradrenaline from the blood stream was not affected by substances which inhibited the action of this enzyme, and there was general agreement that it was not the main agent for removing noradrenaline.

In 1953 the alkaloid reserpine was isolated from the plant *Rauwolfia serpentaria*. When administered to monkeys and to dogs it was observed to have a tranquillizing action. Three years later reserpine was found to reduce the amount of noradrenaline in certain parts of the brain, notably the hypothalamus [40], and to reduce the amounts of adrenaline and noradrenaline in the adrenal medulla [41]. Later it was shown that in animals treated with reserpine the amount of noradrenaline in the heart and blood vessels declined to zero. It had been known for some years that the noradrenaline which could be extracted from the heart and from other organs with a sympathetic innervation must be present within the terminations of the postganglionic fibres, because when these nerves degenerated, the noradrenaline present in the organ disappeared [42]. Thus the administration of reserpine had the effect of removing the noradrenaline from the sympathetic nerve terminals in the course of some hours. A maximal dose removed it in the course of about five hours.

Uptake in the dog. Much work has been done in the last eight years on the uptake of catechol amines and other amines by sympathetic postganglionic fibres. The first demonstrations of uptake were made in 1933 by Burn [137] in the sympathetic nerves supplying the vessels of the dog hind leg. He perfused the vessels with blood after leaving them for 40 min. without a circulation while he prepared the lungs. When the perfusion began, the tone in the hind leg vessels was low and was raised to normal by adding adrenaline drop by drop to the blood reservoir.

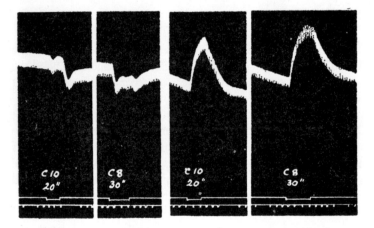

FIG. 7.1. Record of pressure in the arterial cannula tied in the femoral artery of a dog during perfusion of the hind leg. The tone was maintained by the addition of adrenaline drop by drop to the venous reservoir. The two panels on the left show the effect of stimulating the lumbar sympathetic chain early in the perfusion. Some vasodilatation was produced. The two panels on the right show the effects of the same stimulations one hour later in the experiment. Constriction was produced as a result of the uptake of adrenaline by the sympathetic nerve endings. (Burn, 1933.)

When the sympathetic fibres were stimulated at this point, vasodilatation was seen (later shown to be due to release of acetylcholine). However, when the experiment was continued for periods of 1 hr. to 2 hrs. the response to sympathetic stimulation changed and became constrictor. See Fig. 7.1. There were also experiments in which sympathetic stimulation produced initially a small constrictor response which was increased as a result of continued addition of adrenaline to the blood reservoir.

In 1958 Burn and Rand [43] perfused the hind legs of dogs previously treated with reserpine. Stimulation of the sympathetic fibres to the vessels again produced vasodilatation, which was abolished by atropine, and stimulation then had no effect. Addition of 0·5 mg. noradrenaline gradually to the blood reservoir caused vasoconstriction which passed off after 30 min., and when it had done so, and when the blood pressure was back to its previous level, stimulation then caused vasoconstriction, indicating that noradrenaline had been taken up by the sympathetic fibres, and was released again when they were stimulated. These observations, and others of a similar kind which were obtained without the use of either a period of anoxia or of reserpine to remove noradrenaline [125], furnished the most direct evidence of the process of uptake in action which has been published so far.

In 1959 Axelrod et al. [49] showed that when ³H-adrenaline (0.1 mg./kg.) was given intravenously to mice, the unchanged ³H-adrenaline disappeared in two phases; there was a rapid metabolism of 70 per cent, but the rest disappeared slowly, due to transfer from the blood to the tissues. Later work showed that the accumulation of noradrenaline in tissues was greater than that of adrenaline, and that the uptake of noradrenaline was greatest in tissues like the heart with a rich sympathetic innervation. Thus when radioactive noradrenaline was injected intravenously into cats, it was selectively taken up by the heart, spleen and adrenal gland [46]. Other observations again showed that when an intravenous infusion of noradrenaline was given to a rat, the amount of noradrenaline which could be extracted from the heart was approximately doubled [47]. These observations established the fact that noradrenaline was taken up from the blood stream by various organs.

Evidence was also obtained that the uptake was by the nerve endings themselves. Thus the effect of sympathetic stimulation was determined in causing vasoconstriction in the perfused vessels of a dog's hind leg. An infusion of noradrenaline was then given at a uniform rate for twenty or thirty minutes. When the direct effect of the noradrenaline had disappeared some time later, the same stimulation was applied again. It caused a greater vasoconstriction than before [125]. Similar evidence was obtained by administering ^{3}H-noradrenaline to cats. Three hours later, the spleen of the cat was perfused with blood from the femoral artery of a donor cat. When the splenic nerves of the first cat were stimulated, ^{3}H-noradrenaline appeared in the venous effluent from the spleen [126]. Both series of experiments provided evidence that noradrenaline was taken up by the sympathetic nerves, since stimulation does not release noradrenaline except from the nerves. Tissues which were denervated, as for example by removal of the superior cervical ganglion, were not able to take up noradrenaline. Similarly the uptake of ^{3}H-noradrenaline was much reduced in tissues of rats and mice injected at birth with antiserum for the nerve growth factor. Finally ^{3}H-noradrenaline was shown to be localized in postganglionic sympathetic terminals in the rat heart by autoradiography [181].

Features of the uptake process. Iversen [154] has shown that the uptake of noradrenaline is maintained against a concentration gradient, and is therefore an active process. In the isolated rat heart perfused with a solution containing as little as 20 ng./ml. of noradrenaline the concentration in the tissue rises to 40 times that in the perfusing fluid, and the concentration in the sympathetic nerve terminals must be far higher.

The uptake process is more rapid for L-noradrenaline than for L-adrenaline, and more rapid for the L-compounds than for the D-compounds.

Reserpine abolishes the capacity of the granules to bind noradrenaline, but does not affect the initial rate of uptake into the fibre. Normally, when reserpine is absent, binding of noradrenaline by granules occurs very quickly and keeps the concentration of noradrenaline low in the axoplasm.

Second process of uptake. In addition to the first process of uptake which is seen in the rat heart perfused with concentrations of noradrenaline or adrenaline up to $0.5\,\mu g./ml.$, there is a second process of uptake which begins above this concentration and is about twelve times more rapid at a concentration of $1.0\,\mu g./ml.$ This process discovered by Iversen [222] and described as Uptake$_2$ is not greater for the L- than for the D-forms, and has a higher affinity for adrenaline than for noradrenaline.

Isolated storage particles. The particles or granules which store noradrenaline can be isolated. Euler and Lishajko [144] studied uptake in granules from the splenic nerves of the ox. The uptake of noradrenaline was readily demonstrated when ATP and Mg^{++} were present even when the concentration of noradrenaline was less than $1\,\mu g./ml.$ The uptake by granules was much less than that observed in the intact tissue.

O-methyl transferase. While a considerable part of noradrenaline circulating in the blood stream is taken up, a smaller proportion of adrenaline is also taken up. This was shown by a study of the fate of ^{3}H-adrenaline in 1959 [49]. However, both noradrenaline and adrenaline are also destroyed in the body, and the first step in this process was shown to be due to the action of an enzyme O-methyl transferase which was discovered by Axelrod [50].

When noradrenaline was administered, the substance 3-methoxy-4-hydroxymandelic acid was observed to appear in the urine. An enzyme was then found in rat liver capable of transferring a $-CH_3$ group (which is provided by S-adenosyl-methionine) to the $-OH$ group in the meta position in the ring.

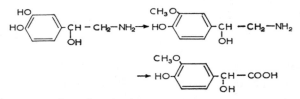

The enzyme effects this change in noradrenaline, adrenaline and other catechols; it was found in rat liver and kidney, and to a smaller extent in other organs, including brain. It was also found in human liver.

Following the formation from noradrenaline of the 3-methoxy compound (which is called normetanephrine), monoamine oxidase removes the amine group, and in this way 3-methoxy-4-hydroxymandelic acid is formed. Similar changes take place in adrenaline, and in other substances such as dopamine and dopa.

Amines which release noradrenaline. When animals have been injected with reserpine 5–18 hours previously and have lost the noradrenaline present in the sympathetic fibres in the heart, blood vessels and other organs, not only does stimulation of postganglionic sympathetic fibres fail to cause its usual effect, but the action of certain sympathomimetic amines is also lost [43]. Three of these amines, which are not catechol amines, have the structures shown. They are

When injected into the vein of a normal anaesthetized animal,

64

these substances cause a rise of blood pressure. When injected into an animal which has received reserpine on the previous day, they no longer cause a rise of blood pressure. However, if the animal which has been treated with reserpine is first given a slow intravenous infusion of noradrenaline, then these substances cause a rise of blood pressure [43]. The action of tyramine was thus restored in the rat, not only by noradrenaline, but also by dopamine, L-dopa, meta-tyrosine and phenylalanine. Apparently all these substances can be taken up into the nerve endings and converted there into noradrenaline. This can be released by tyramine. From these findings the conclusion was drawn that tyramine, ephedrine and amphetamine act by releasing noradrenaline.

On the blood pressure dopamine still acts in the reserpine-treated cat, so that here dopamine acts directly. But when the store of noradrenaline is removed from the iris by dropping guanethidine into the conjunctival sac for 3 or 4 days, then dopamine has no dilator effect on the pupil, though phenylephrine still causes dilatation. Phenylephrine acts directly like noradrenaline.

The proof that these substances release noradrenaline was obtained by making experiments on the isolated rabbit heart perfused through the aorta. When some form of Ringer's solution runs into the aorta, it closes the aortic valves, so that the solution does not enter the left ventricle; instead it enters the coronary arteries and finds its way out into the right atrium mainly through the coronary sinus. A heart perfused in this way continues to beat for many hours. In the fluid leaving the heart there was found a small amount of noradrenaline. If tyramine was added to the fluid entering the heart, the amount of noradrenaline leaving the heart was greatly increased, until, for example, seven times as much came out [52].

If the splenic nerves of cattle are taken, they can be homogenized and centrifuged. By high speed centrifugation in a sucrose density gradient it is possible to isolate a layer containing granules which are very rich in noradrenaline [53]. These granules also contain adenosine triphosphate, which is present in an amount bearing a fixed relation to the amount of noradrenaline. The conclusion has been drawn that noradrenaline and ATP are chemically combined in the granules. When the granules were incubated in the presence of oxygen at a temperature of $37°C$, they liberated noradrenaline at a slow rate. When tyramine was added to the suspension of granules, the amount of noradrenaline liberated was greatly increased, up to $2\frac{1}{2}$ times. It appeared that tyramine, being a stronger base than noradrenaline, entered the granules and displaced the noradrenaline from its combination with adenosine triphosphate [54]. Ephedrine and amphetamine acted in the same way as tyramine. Others have confirmed these results [144, 145].

The action of tyramine is therefore indirect and unlike that of noradrenaline. Tyramine does not cause vasoconstriction itself, but enters the postganglionic sympathetic fibres and liberates noradrenaline from them.

When reserpine was given and the amount of noradrenaline present in the heart was examined, the action of tyramine on the heart rate did not decline until the amount of noradrenaline had fallen to about 10 per cent of its normal value. Then as the amount of noradrenaline diminished further, the effect of tyramine diminished rapidly until it was completely absent. When the heart, depleted of noradrenaline and unresponsive to tyramine, was exposed to noradrenaline so that noradrenaline was taken up again, the action of tyramine reappeared when the amount of noradrenaline present in the heart was not more than 2 per cent of the amount normally present [55].

The effect of denervation. Since the noradrenaline present in an organ like the heart is contained in the terminations of the sympathetic fibres, it follows that when the sympathetic fibres degenerate, the organ must lose most of its noradrenaline; this was shown by Euler and Purkhold [42] in 1951. The denervated organ should therefore behave towards sympathomimetic amines as the organ behaves in an animal treated with reserpine. This is what has been observed. Thus tyramine and ephedrine were found to have little or no action on the iris and on the vessels of the cat's foreleg after degeneration of the sympathetic fibres [56].

On the other hand adrenaline was shown to have a greater action on the denervated iris [57], and recently noradrenaline has been shown to have a greater action on denervated arteries [58], as it has on several other denervated tissues. These results correspond with the majority of observations concerning the action of noradrenaline and adrenaline on organs in animals treated with reserpine. On the whole these organs give a greater response to noradrenaline than do the organs from normal animals, but there are exceptions, notably the nictitating membrane in the spinal cat and the iris of the cat. An explanation of these exceptions may be that when reserpine is injected, not only does it liberate noradrenaline from its stores in sympathetic nerve endings, but it attaches itself to the effector sites which are stimulated by noradrenaline and blocks them. This has been demonstrated in the isolated atria of the rabbit heart [59].

However, in the main it is true that organs which are taken from animals treated with reserpine respond to sympathomimetic amines in the same way as do denervated organs. The response of both is diminished to amines which act by liberating noradrenaline, while the response of both is increased to noradrenaline and adrenaline.

Amphetamine. The properties of amphetamine are far from being fully understood. It is well known to prevent sleepiness and to make a man able to work without fatigue for much longer than usual. Amphetamine has been found valuable for treating oedema of the legs in women who have no cardiac weakness [307]. In those who take it there is an increase in fluorogenic corticosteroids specially marked in the evening. Reinert [269] has shown that amphetamine produces depolarization and block in the cat's superior cervical ganglion identical to that seen after nicotine. He thinks that this nicotinic action of amphetamine may be the mode of action of its central stimulating properties.

Action of monoamine oxidase. Although it is true that monoamine oxidase appears to play a relatively unimportant part in the destruction of noradrenaline, its action is evident so far as amines like tyramine and ephedrine are concerned. Ephedrine contains a $-CH_3$ group on the carbon atom next to the amine group in the side-chain, and for this reason cannot be destroyed by amine oxidase. Amphetamine resembles ephedrine in this respect. Tyramine, however, has no such group and it is an excellent substrate for monoamine oxidase. The difference is seen very well in the heart-lung preparation of the dog when the effect of these amines on the heart rate is examined. Tyramine in the amount of 1 mg. produces a rise in the rate of relatively short duration. The rate returns to the initial rate in about twenty minutes. Ephedrine and amphetamine, however, cause a rise in the heart rate which is maintained for two or three hours, or even longer. Tyramine is shortlived in action because it is destroyed by monoamine oxidase. Ephedrine and amphetamine are prolonged in action because they are not destroyed by monoamine oxidase [61].

Various amines have been synthesized by pharmaceutical firms for use in raising the blood pressure. Some of them are

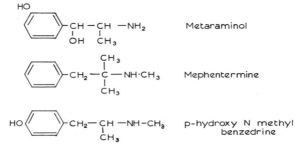

Some of these amines have both a direct action like noradrenaline and an indirect action like tyramine. Metaraminol is one of these; it has an –OH group on the carbon atom in the side-chain which is next to the benzene ring; this gives it a direct action, borne out by the fact that it has a good pressor action in the animal treated with reserpine. Metaraminol, like the other amines, has a –CH₃ group on the carbon atom next to the amine group; this group prevents its destruction by monoamine oxidase. The other two substances have no direct action, but cause a rise in pressure by releasing noradrenaline.

Monoamine oxidase inhibitors. Substances which inhibit the action of monoamine oxidase are used in psychiatry to relieve depression. Such substances include iproniazid, nialamide, phenelzine and tranylcypromine. The structure of this last is

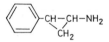

The effectiveness of these compounds suggests that depression may be due to a diminution of the concentration of amines in the brain.

Patients who are treated with inhibitors become sensitive to cheese and to beans. Cheese contains tyramine formed from tyrosine. Ordinarily when cheese is eaten the tyramine is destroyed by monoamine oxidase. But when an inhibitor of this enzyme is given the tyramine is not destroyed and may cause a large rise of blood pressure. Intracranial haemorrhage has occurred as a result [155, 156]. Broad beans contain dopa in their pods, and if they are sliced and cooked whole, or if bean meal is prepared, then dopa is eaten and dopamine is formed from it. This is not destroyed by monoamine oxidase in the presence of an inhibitor, and is probably converted to noradrenaline. Consumption of ½ lb. whole cooked broad beans has raised the blood pressure from 165 to 262 mm. in a patient treated with 37 mg. pargyline daily. This effect of pargyline was confirmed in volunteers [157].

Precursors of noradrenaline. In the cat treated with reserpine to deplete the sympathetic terminals of noradrenaline, tyramine was found to have very little action on the blood pressure. However, its power to raise the blood pressure was restored by a slow intravenous infusion of noradrenaline, and also by an infusion of one of the precursors of noradrenaline, namely dopamine, or L-dopa or phenylalanine [44]. It was supposed that these precursors were taken up into sympathetic fibres, where they were converted to noradrenaline. Tyramine was then able to cause a rise of blood pressure again by releasing noradrenaline.

Formation of false transmitters. Not only is noradrenaline formed in sympathetic fibres by uptake of its precursors, but other compounds may be formed also. Thus the compound α-methyl dopa is used in the treatment of high blood pressure. When administered to man it is taken up by sympathetic fibres and converted to α-methyl noradrenaline. This compound is stored in the granules and dilutes the store of noradrenaline. Sympathetic impulses then release both substances and since α-methyl noradrenaline is less active than noradrenaline, the physiological response to a given stimulation of the fibres is less than it was. The compound α-methyl noradrenaline has been called a false transmitter [124]. The release of α-methyl noradrenaline in response to sympathetic stimulation was first demonstrated by Muscholl and Maître [270] in the isolated rabbit heart.

In the body the amino acid tyrosine is partly converted to tyramine by decarboxylation, but normally tyramine is destroyed by monoamine oxidase. Patients who are given substances which inhibit the action of this enzyme do not destroy tyramine, and this enters sympathetic fibres (where the monoamine oxidase is also inhibited) and is there converted to octopamine. This is effected by hydroxylation of the carbon atom adjacent to the benzene ring. (Octopamine was so called because it was first found by Erspamer in the posterior salivary gland of the octopus.) The octopamine formed in the sympathetic fibre is then released by sympathetic impulses, and is another example of a false transmitter [223]. This is believed to be the mode of action of inhibitors of monoamine oxidase in causing a fall of blood pressure (See also 271).

CHAPTER 8

SUBSTANCES WHICH PREVENT
THE UPTAKE OF NORADRENALINE.
THE ACTION OF COCAINE

The action of cocaine. That postganglionic sympathetic fibres take up noradrenaline from the blood stream is a new conception of considerable importance. Whether there are substances normally present in the body which can diminish or prevent this uptake is unknown, but there are substances not normally present which have this action. It is best established for cocaine, but there is evidence that it is possessed by other substances as well. Studies made with cocaine have revealed new features of the activity of the sympathetic nerve endings which have a physiological importance for the control of vascular tone.

Cocaine is an alkaloid present in coca leaves. These leaves are commonly chewed by those who work in the silver mines of the Andes, where mining is carried on at high altitudes. The oxygen tension there is low. The effect of chewing the leaves is that cocaine is absorbed, and chewing is found to increase the working capacity of the miners. The social problem created by the chewing of coca leaves has been much discussed. Some have argued that the habit has persisted because the mine-owners have paid too low wages, and that the workers have been able to afford only a limited diet of poor quality. However, the alkaloid cocaine present in coca leaves has actions in the body which are compatible with the view that an increase in working capacity is produced by chewing the leaves. What is of special interest is that the changes produced by cocaine are both central and peripheral.

The effect of cocaine on sympathomimetic amines. As long ago as 1910 it was shown that after the injection of cocaine into an anaesthetized animal, the rise of blood pressure caused by an intravenous injection of a given amount of adrenaline was increased. Not only did the blood pressure rise to a greater height than before, but the return of the blood pressure to normal was delayed [62]. Several years later it was observed that the injection of cocaine had the opposite effect on the rise of blood pressure caused by tyramine [63] or by ephedrine [64]. An injection of cocaine might not only diminish the rise caused by tyramine or by ephedrine, but might abolish it altogether.

Thus the effect of cocaine was to produce a condition very like that which was recently seen to be produced in an animal injected with reserpine. The rise of blood pressure caused by adrenaline was increased, and that caused by tyramine was decreased both when reserpine was given several hours previously, and also immediately after the giving of cocaine. The action of reserpine was due to the slow discharge of noradrenaline from the sympathetic nerve endings. To what was the action of cocaine due?

TABLE 8.1.

Effect of cocaine on concentration of noradrenaline in the plasma after the injection of 25 μg./kg. noradrenaline
(Trendelenburg, 65)

	Noradrenaline concentration in plasma (μg./ml.)		
	1 *min.*	2 *min.*	3 *min.*
Control	74·5	25·8	15·2
Cocaine, 2·5 mg./kg.	133·1	65·7	42·1
,, 5·0 ,,	144·2	73·9	56·0

The first step in explanation was a demonstration that when noradrenaline was injected into a spinal cat, the rate at which it disappeared from the blood plasma was much slower in the presence of cocaine [65]. In a series of cats a certain dose of noradrenaline was injected, and blood was taken after 1 minute, 2 minutes and 3 minutes to determine the amount present in the plasma. Cocaine was given and the same dose of noradrenaline was injected again; the amount found in the plasma was then greater after each sampling as shown in Table 8.1. After cocaine was injected in the amount of 5 mg./kg., the noradrenaline present in the plasma was twice as great at the end of 1 minute, and more than three times as great at the end of 3 minutes. The rise of blood pressure caused by noradrenaline in the presence of cocaine was also greater in height and duration. The half-life of noradrenaline in the plasma agreed fairly well with the half time of the return of the blood pressure to normal both before and after cocaine. Hence the delay in disappearance of noradrenaline from the plasma fully accounted for the increased response of the blood pressure in the presence of cocaine.

Effect of cocaine on uptake. These results suggested that the delay in the removal of noradrenaline from the plasma in the presence of cocaine might be explained by a diminished uptake of noradrenaline. It seemed possible that the passage of noradrenaline into the sympathetic nerve endings might be prevented by cocaine. This suggestion was shown to be correct by infusing noradrenaline into pithed rats and measuring the uptake by the heart and spleen. It was observed that the noradrenaline which was infused (20 μg.) increased the amount of noradrenaline in the heart by 78 per cent, and increased the amount of noradrenaline in the spleen by 79 per cent. When (in other experiments) the rats were previously given cocaine, the increase in the heart was only 25 per cent, and in the spleen only 15 per cent. The results are shown in Table 8.2 [66].

A study was also made of the relation between the increase in the pressor response to noradrenaline which cocaine produced, and the amount taken up by the heart. In those rats in which cocaine increased the pressor response greatly, the amount taken up was small, and in those in which it increased the pressor

TABLE 8.2.

Cocaine prevents uptake of noradrenaline
(Muscholl, 66)

Cocaine mg./kg.	Noradrenaline infused in 20 min.	Noradrenaline µg./g.	
		Heart	Spleen
—	—	0·59	0·19
—	20 µg.	1·05	0·34
10	20 ,,	0·85	0·26
20	20 ,,	0·74	0·22

response less, the amount taken up was greater. The results showed that when noradrenaline was introduced into the blood, part of it was taken up by sympathetic nerve endings without having any effect; only that part which was not taken up had an action on blood pressure and other organs. The observation [69] that cocaine did not increase the action of noradrenaline on the nictitating membrane when this had been denervated for 10 days, supported the view that cocaine prevented uptake into sympathetic nerves.

The assumption could then be made that if cocaine prevented the uptake of noradrenaline, it would also prevent the uptake of tyramine. Both substances are amines of the same general structure. Tyramine differs from noradrenaline in that outside the sympathetic nerve fibre it has little or no action. The action of tyramine begins when it enters the nerve fibre and liberates noradrenaline. If cocaine prevents the entry of tyramine in the same way as it prevents the entry of noradrenaline, it would abolish the action of tyramine.

The activity of sympathetic nerve endings. Observations on the rate of the isolated atria of the rabbit heart showed that when they were suspended in a modified Ringer's solution at a given temperature, the rate of beating of different atria varied, but the mean rate was 145 beats per minute. It appeared that the noradrenaline present within the terminations of the sympathetic fibres contributed to this rate, for when atria from rabbits injected with reserpine on the previous day were examined, atria from which noradrenaline was absent, it was observed that the mean rate was lower, being 112 beats per minute. This figure was significantly different from the mean rate of atria from normal rabbits [67]. The difference suggested that in the normal atria there was a continuous liberation of noradrenaline from the postganglionic terminations in the atria, this liberation being sufficient to raise the pacemaker rate from 112 to 145.

When cocaine was added to the bath in which the normal atria were suspended, the atrial rate rose. Thus in one experiment the addition of cocaine hydrochloride to make a concentration of 5×10^{-6}g./ml., raised the rate by 18 beats per minute [68]. This rise might be explained by supposing that some of the noradrenaline which was released from the sympathetic nerve endings was normally reabsorbed without exerting any action. If in the presence of cocaine this reabsorption was prevented, the whole of the noradrenaline which was released would then act on the pacemaker.

Thus the picture is suggested of a situation where the postganglionic sympathetic fibre, even in the absence of impulses passing along the fibre, is constantly releasing a small amount of noradrenaline, part of which is reabsorbed and part of which exerts an action. If this is true of sympathetic nerve endings in the atria, it may be true of all sympathetic nerve endings throughout the body, and the tone of the blood vessels, for example, may be in part determined by this continual release. Certainly in the spinal cat, in which the flow of impulses along the nerves to the arteries must be small, the injection of cocaine into the muscles of the cat in the amount of 3 mg./kg., is followed by a rise in the blood pressure level, which is maintained about 20 mm. higher than previously. There is also a rise in the tone of the normally innervated nictitating membrane, though none in that of the denervated membrane [69].

Action of cocaine on sympathetic stimulation. The view that cocaine blocks the uptake not only of noradrenaline which is injected into the blood stream, but also of noradrenaline which is spontaneously released by the unstimulated sympathetic nerve ending, is supported by the effect of cocaine on the response to stimulation of postganglionic fibres. When the fibres to the nictitating membrane were stimulated, the response was increased by the injection of cocaine [65] and when the accelerator fibres to the isolated atria of the heart were stimulated the increase in rate was greater in the presence of cocaine [68].

The action of cocaine in skeletal muscle. The consequence of the action of cocaine in blocking uptake of noradrenaline can be observed in skeletal muscle. When the gastrocnemius of the cat perfused with blood by a pump was stimulated intermittently through the sciatic nerve by break induction shocks (at the rate of 32/sec. applied for 0·13 second, the interval between each application being 0·39/sec.), the muscle contractions developed a tension of about 4 kg. When 2 mg. cocaine was injected into the perfusing blood, the tension increased to 5 kg. In the absence of cocaine the tension was similarly increased by the injection of 4 μg. adrenaline, and in the presence of cocaine the injection of 4 μg. adrenaline produced a much greater increase [70].

It is probable that the increase in tension resulting from the injection of adrenaline is explained by an increase in the percentage of impulses transmitted to the muscle. When the motor nerves are stimulated repeatedly the percentage of impulses which are transmitted falls, so that perhaps only 60 per cent are effective. Adrenaline has been shown to restore this percentage to 100 [28].

When the sciatic nerve is stimulated, not only motor fibres but also sympathetic fibres are involved, and the noradrenaline released by sympathetic stimulation will help to maintain the percentage of impulses which are transmitted. Some of the noradrenaline will, however, be reabsorbed and have no action. The effect of cocaine will then be to stop the reabsorption, so that all the noradrenaline then is available to increase the percentage of impulses transmitted.

In the same way, when adrenaline is injected, some of it is absorbed into sympathetic nerve endings and some acts on receptors. After the injection of cocaine none of the adrenaline is absorbed and all of it acts on receptors. Thus the effect of cocaine in preventing the uptake of adrenaline and of noradrenaline by sympathetic nerve fibres can explain its effect in increasing the tension developed by skeletal muscle when the sciatic nerve is stimulated repeatedly over long periods of time.

The central action of cocaine. The action of cocaine in blocking uptake of noradrenaline seems not to be confined to peripheral structures but to be evident within the central nervous system itself. It is, of course, well known that cocaine has an action on the central nervous system, since cocaine is a drug of addiction and is generally taken like snuff. Cocaine causes excitement and a feeling of wellbeing. It increases conversational powers and heightens the imagination. It may produce pleasing hallucinations. These are the credit items in the balance sheet, but there are debit items as well which result from frequent use. Thus the nasal mucous membranes with which cocaine comes in contact suffer because of the vasoconstriction which the cocaine causes; this results in ulceration. More serious, however, are the effects on personality, which becomes debased. The addict comes to believe that he is persecuted, and carries weapons to defend himself. He suffers physically from loss of appetite and inability to sleep. The investigations into the chewing of coca leaves have been undertaken because of the bad effects which the chewing produces.

Thus an investigation has been made into the effects of cocaine on mice. Mice do not keep still, but are constantly moving, and by putting them in a suitably designed cage in which their movements interfere with the light shining on a photocell, their activity over periods of time can be measured. If the mice are injected with reserpine, in the course of a few hours they become tranquil and their activity stops. This arrest of activity seems to be due to the disappearance of noradrenaline from the brain, in particular from the hypothalamus, because the activity can be restored by giving the mice L-dopa, which is an amino-acid from which dopamine and then noradrenaline are formed. L-dopa, being an amino-acid and not an amine, can pass the blood brain barrier and enter the brain. It is there decarboxylated to form dopamine, and the dopamine is oxidized to form noradrenaline.

Now when cocaine is given to normal mice, their activity increases, and the effect of cocaine can be measured. If, however, the mice are treated with reserpine and are inactive, the giving of cocaine does not restore their activity. This indicates that the action of cocaine in normal mice depends on the presence of noradrenaline. Further evidence is provided by giving L-dopa to the mice which have been treated with reserpine, giving it in a small amount which by itself is insufficient to restore the activity of the mice. If cocaine is then given, it soon restores the normal activity. This also indicates that the action of cocaine in normal mice depends on the presence of noradrenaline [72].

In peripheral tissues we have seen that the effect of cocaine is due to an effect at sympathetic nerve endings. These endings are continually releasing noradrenaline, some of which is taken up again by the endings and some of which produces a physiological effect, such as raising the rate at which the pacemaker discharges impulses in the atria. Cocaine prevents the uptake, and therefore the amount of noradrenaline available to produce a physiological effect is increased. It is possible that the central effects produced by cocaine are produced by exactly the same mechanism as the peripheral effects. The central effects of excitement and of euphoria may be due to a rise in the concentration of free noradrenaline in the hypothalamus and in other parts of the brain, due to interference with uptake.

Other substances which block uptake. A quantitative study has been made [158] of the uptake of noradrenaline when perfused through the isolated rabbit heart. When noradrenaline alone was infused about 60 per cent was recovered in the perfusate. In the presence of cocaine, or of guanethidine, the amount recovered in the perfusate was 90 per cent or more, so that these agents blocked uptake as also did the beta-blocking agents dichloroisoprenaline and pronethalol.

Other observations have been made in the perfused spleen [159] in which the amount of noradrenaline recovered in the perfusate was as little as 29 per cent. When cocaine or phenoxybenzamine was present the recovery was high, being 82 per cent, and a similar figure was obtained when noradrenaline alone was perfused through spleens in which the nerves had degenerated. Other antiadrenaline agents as well as phenoxybenzamine, namely Hydergine and phentolamine, increased the percentage of noradrenaline recovered from 29 per cent to 62 per cent.

Many sympathomimetic amines have been shown by Burgen and Iversen [160] to compete with noradrenaline for uptake into the isolated rat heart, and thus to block the uptake of noradrenaline. Thus D-amphetamine is very powerful in this respect, and in general those substances having a $-CH_3$ group on the carbon atom next to the amine group are powerful. On the other hand the presence of an –OH group on the carbon atom next to the benzene ring has the opposite effect. Hence amphetamine is more powerful than phenylethylamine, but phenylethylamine is more powerful than phenylethanolamine.

A study has also been made of the uptake, not of noradrenaline, but of ^{3}H-metaraminol into the mouse heart. In order to test substances for their power to block uptake, they were given to the mice in a dose of 10 mg./kg. five minutes before the ^{3}H-metaraminol was given. Cocaine was found to reduce the uptake to 46 per cent of the control value, while amitriptyline reduced it to 32 per cent, and imipramine reduced it to 25 per cent of the control value. These two substances are used in psychiatry to elevate the mood of those suffering from depression. They may act in the brain like cocaine [193].

CHAPTER 9

TRANSMITTERS IN THE BRAIN

Acetylcholine. The identification of transmitters in the brain is clearly much more difficult than in the peripheral nervous system, and the progress which has been made, in view of the uncertainty of the direction and destination of the nerve fibres, is remarkable. The first substance shown to act as a transmitter is acetylcholine. That it is released from the surface of the brain was discovered by MacIntosh and Oborin in 1953. Their method was to make a hole in the dura, and to stand a small glass tube with open ends upright on the surface. They put Ringer containing the anticholinesterase physostigmine in the tube, and found that in course of time acetylcholine accumulated in the solution. The amount was much less in the animal anaesthetized with chloralose. Later it was found that if atropine was given to the animal, the amount of acetylcholine released was much greater. A simple explanation of this is that normally the acetylcholine is released to act on receptors, and in acting on these receptors the acetylcholine is destroyed. Atropine blocks these receptors so that the acetylcholine is not destroyed and thus more of it accumulates in the presence of the physostigmine.

A part of the brain in which a special study of the release of acetylcholine has been made is the caudate nucleus. Studies have been made by the use of a 'push–pull' cannula. This consists of an inner needle surrounded by an outer needle. Fluid is driven into a small area of tissue through the inner needle and sucked out through the outer needle. With this device it was observed that stimulation of a small area of the frontal cortex of a cat caused release of acetylcholine from the caudate nucleus. A similar release was observed on stimulation of one of the thalamic nuclei.

Another method of studying the release in the caudate nucleus is by superfusing the nucleus. This can be done by perfusing the anterior horn of the lateral ventricle of a cat, using an artificial cerebrospinal fluid for perfusing. When an anticholinesterase (neostigmine) is added to the fluid, acetylcholine begins to appear in the perfusate, and steadily rises in concentration as the anaesthesia of the cat gets less. Superimposed on this rising basal release, Portig and Vogt found an additional release in response to four different stimuli. These were electrical stimulation of the cat's paws, stimulation of the sciatic nerves, stimulation of the opposite caudate nucleus, and finally stimulation by noise. They also observed a rise when they placed electrodes into the substantia nigra. Evidently there are many pathways to the caudate nucleus, and at the end of these pathways they arrive at a place where the transmission is effected by the release of acetylcholine. If the cholinesterase is inhibited by neostigmine, then some of the liberated acetylcholine finds its way into the perfusing fluid. Cholinergic neurones are not to be found everywhere in the brain, and some regions contain many more than others, as was shown by the distribution of the enzyme choline acetyltransferase which synthesizes acetylcholine. The presence of these neurones has also been demonstrated by staining for acetylcholinesterase, making lesions to indicate the direction in which the fibres travelled. When an axon is severed, the enzyme accumulates on the side of the cut connected to the cell body.

The ascending reticular formation. This latter method led to the conclusion that the ascending reticular activating system consists mainly of cholinergic neurones, and this is supported by the evidence that anticholinesterases cause arousal, as shown by

83

fast waves and asynchrony in the electrocorticogram. Atropine abolishes this effect and causes slow waves.

Noradrenaline. A study of the distribution of noradrenaline in the brain was first made by Vogt in 1954. She found the highest concentration to be in the hypothalamus, and slightly lower concentrations in the midbrain and in the medulla. Fluorescence microscopy has revealed that the noradrenaline is present in neurones which have origin in the cells of the midbrain, and many of the neurones terminate in the hypothalamus.

Release of noradrenaline by stimulation has recently been demonstrated by Philippu, Heyd and Burger [273]. They injected labelled noradrenaline into the third ventricle, and after 4 hours placed a cannula in the aqueduct of Sylvius and perfused the ventricle with artificial cerebrospinal fluid. In this way they perfused the hypothalamus. During the perfusion noradrenaline and its metabolites (such as 3-methoxy, 4-hydroxymandelic acid) were released, and when the rate of release had been determined, studies were made of the effects of (1) electrical stimulation, (2) acetylcholine and (3) calcium ions.

Electrical stimulation of the nucleus anterior medialis, and also of the nuclei posterior and ventro-medialis increased the release of noradrenaline and its metabolites. The important observation was made that the perfusion of the third ventricle with acetylcholine increased the release of noradrenaline from the hypothalamus, and that this effect of acetylcholine was dependent on the presence of calcium. When calcium was absent, acetylcholine had no effect. Finally the authors were able to show that when calcium was removed altogether by perfusion of the ventricle with EDTA for 1 hour, followed by perfusion with calcium-free solution, then perfusion with a solution containing calcium ions increased the release of noradrenaline.

These results, concerning the release of noradrenaline from

84

the hypothalamus, resemble those obtained by Douglas and Rubin [170] in the adrenal medulla; they also resemble those obtained by Burn and Gibbons [276] in the isolated atria of the rabbit, in which (in the presence of hyoscine) the percentage increase in rate caused by acetylcholine was proportional to the calcium concentration. Thus in the hypothalamus the release of noradrenaline by electrical stimulation may be due, as it is in the adrenal gland and in the sympathetic postganglionic fibre, to the initial release of acetylcholine, which then makes the membrane which surrounds the granules containing noradrenaline permeable to calcium. Calcium then passes through the membrane and releases noradrenaline.

Further information on this will be obtained when electrical stimulation is applied at a frequency of 1 cps rather than (as in the experiments of Philippu *et al.*) at a frequency of 40 cps. For at 1 cps, the presence of an anticholinesterase may greatly increase the response to stimulation [274].

Action of nicotine. In keeping with this work of Philippu *et al.* is the finding of G. H. Hall and D. M. Turner that when labelled noradrenaline is injected into the 3rd ventricle and then, 1 hour later, the ventricle is perfused with artificial cerebrospinal fluid, the intravenous injection of 2 μg./kg. nicotine every 30 sec. for 30 min., or the intraventricular perfusion of 2 μg./ml. of nicotine for 30 min. causes an increase in the amount of labelled noradrenaline in the perfusate.

Action of amphetamine. D-amphetamine has a simliar effect to that of nicotine [272]. When d-amphetamine was added to the fluid perfusing the cat ventricle in a concentration of 100 μg./ml., the ventricle having previously received an injection of tritiated noradrenaline, during the period in which d-amphetamine was present in the perfusate, there was a threefold increase in the release of noradrenaline. Reinert [269] has previously shown that nicotine and amphetamine have well-marked properties in common, and the effect of amphetamine may therefore be described as a nicotine-like effect.

Dopamine in the caudate nucleus

Dopamine. In 1959 Carlsson discovered that there was much dopamine in the corpus striatum, about 10 μg./g., while there was almost no noradrenaline. Then in the following year Ehringer and Hornykiewicz found that, in the caudate nucleus and putamen of patients who had died from Parkinson's disease, the amount of dopamine was only 10 per cent of the normal value, and also that the same was true of homovanillic acid, the main metabolite of dopamine. The work of Oscar and Cécile Vogt had shown that the histological changes in the striatum were few in patients with Parkinson's disease, despite the presence of so little dopamine, and the picture was in striking contrast with the atrophy of the striatum in Huntington's chorea, in which the dopamine concentration was normal.

The first suggestion that the *substantia nigra* was the site of the causative lesion in Parkinson's disease came from Trétiakoff in 1919, and this was confirmed by Hassler in 1938 who found a correlation between the destruction of the *substantia nigra* and the signs of the disease. Thus there was reason for thinking that there was a tract of nerve fibres originating in the *substantia nigra* and terminating in the caudate nucleus where dopamine was liberated as the transmitter. Experimental evidence for this view was first obtained by making lesions in the midbrain of monkeys, the lesions including the *substantia nigra*, as a result of which a lowered content of dopamine was found chemically in the tissue of the striatum.

Release of dopamine. The first evidence of release of dopamine came from McLennan who placed electrodes in the *substantia nigra* and obtained release of dopamine on stimulation from the outflow of a push–pull cannula placed in the putamen. However Portig and Vogt perfused the cerebral ventricle of cats, and tested the effluent for dopamine when they stimulated the *substantia nigra*. They observed a very small release. They then turned their attention to homovanillic acid, the main metabolite of dopamine, and were much more successful. The homovanillic acid formed in the striatum entered the ventricular perfusate and was then estimated fluorimetrically. There was in most experiments an increase in the stimulation period of 30–100 ng. per 30 min. and it often lasted over an hour.

Effects of tranquillizing drugs. Another interesting development of the dopamine story turns on the observation that drugs such as chlorpromazine, which are useful in treating schizophrenia, produce the symptoms of Parkinson's disease in some patients. The curious observation has been made that these drugs produce an accumulation of homovanillic acid in the striatum of rabbits, though there is no diminution in the amount of dopamine. Thus these drugs cause an increase in the turnover of dopamine. The effect on the homovanillic acid is seen only when the substances which cause Parkinsonism are tested. Thus a comparison was made of chlorpromazine, trifluoperazine, thioproperazine and thioridazine, of which the first three cause Parkinson symptoms, while thioridazine does not. In the course of 14 days when given to cats once a day, the first three substances caused increases of 60 per cent, 70 per cent and 120 per cent in the homovanillic acid in the caudate nucleus, while the fourth substance caused no increase.

The comparison between chlorpromazine and haloperidol was the most striking. In man, haloperidol is about 50 times as potent as chlorpromazine for treating psychoses and for producing Parkinson symptoms, and the same ratio of potency was observed for the effect on dopamine concentration in the mouse striatum and for the rise in homovanillic acid. However the

87

problem remains why Parkinson's disease occurs when there is a loss of dopamine from the striatum in man, but the symptoms of Parkinsonism appear when drugs are given which increase the turnover of dopamine without reducing its amount.

There is a further point of interest for the present writer. He believes that it has been clearly demonstrated that the release of noradrenaline from the sympathetic postganglionic fibre is effected by the action of acetylcholine. One of the observations which has been made is that when all noradrenaline is removed by reserpine, stimulation of the splenic nerves in the cat releases acetylcholine. This has also been observed in the rabbit heart and other organs. It looks as though acetylcholine is normally used in releasing noradrenaline, but when there is none to release, the acetylcholine then acts on acetylcholine receptors dilating the spleen or slowing the heart. It is possible that the release of dopamine from the nigro-striatal terminations is also accomplished by acetylcholine, and if so, when the disease of Parkinsonism has reduced the dopamine, then effects due to acetylcholine would be seen which normally are not. In fact there are effects of this kind, and they are abolished or diminished by giving atropine or hyoscine as part of the treatment of Parkinsonism. The fact that tubocurarine has been found to release dopamine from the superfused caudate nucleus may not be unconnected with a release of dopamine by acetylcholine. (For references to many of the observations described in the foregoing account, the reader should consult the lecture by Dr. Marthe Vogt which is published in the *British J. Pharmacology* (1969) **37,** 325–37.)

GABA (gamma-aminobutyric acid) is an amino-acid which has been suggested to be a transmitter liberated by inhibitory neurones in the brain. The idea was based on its distribution and metabolism, its release from nervous tissue when inhibitory neurones were active, and the fact that, when administered by microelectrophoresis, it hyperpolarized neurones in Deiter's nucleus and the cerebral cortex. But now Curtis *et al.* [275] have given much stronger support to the idea by finding that *Bicucullin*, an alkaloid obtained from a species of Corydalis, blocks the inhibitory effect of Gaba on central neurones and reduces the inhibition (the strychnine-resistant inhibition) of cortical pyramidal and cerebellar Purkinje cells. This discovery of an agent which blocks the action of Gaba, makes it far more likely that Gaba is in fact a transmitter of inhibitory impulses.

Glycine an inhibitor in the spinal cord. In the spinal cord strychnine is an agent which suppresses postsynaptic inhibition, and which is a competitive antagonist of glycine, another amino-acid thought to be released as an inhibitory transmitter from spinal neurones. But strychnine does not suppress the inhibitory effect of Gaba in neurones in the brain. Curtis therefore studied the essential features of the strychnine molecule which could provide the key to its interaction with glycine receptors, and having done so examined several convulsant isoquinoline alkaloids which might combine with Gaba receptors. Thus he found bicucullin, which is a phthalide isoquinoline.

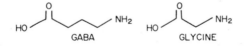

CHAPTER 10

PROPERTIES OF 5-HYDROXYTRYPTAMINE

The importance of 5-hydroxytryptamine, or 5-HT, which was first found to be the vasoconstrictor substance in serum, and therefore called serotonin, and later found in argentaffin cells in the intestine, is increasingly related to the nervous system, both central and peripheral. In the medulla and pons 5-HT is found in the cells of the midline (or raphe) nuclei, the terminals being distributed in the hypothalamus and the brain stem. Attempts have been made to stimulate the raphe nuclei, whilst collecting fluid in cups on the sigmoid gyrus [277]; an increase in 5-HT was indeed obtained but the amounts were very small. Other attempts at stimulation during perfusion of the anterior horn of a lateral ventricle have also failed to produce satisfactory amounts.

Important observations have been made by Jouvet and Renault [278] as a result of making surgical lesions in the raphe nuclei. They found that these lesions prevented sleep in cats and rats. They confirmed their results by using p-chlorphenylal-anine, which inhibits tryptophan hydroxylase and so prevents 5-HT formation. Sleep was again impossible.

It was also found [279] that when this substance is given, rats suffer from hyperalgesia, and only very large doses of morphine can produce analgesia. When the 5-HT in the mouse brain is increased, then the reverse is seen and the toxicity of pethidine increases in proportion to the increase.

Another effect of p-chlorphenylalanine which was recorded by Shillito was that when it was given to young male rats they groomed one another so persistently that they became bald unless they were separated. In adult rats frequent mounting was seen. The effect on males was abolished by atropine. There was no obvious effect on females. All signs of abnormal behaviour were absent if 5-hydroxytryptophan was given shortly before the observations, so the strange behaviour was due to the absence of 5-HT.

5-HT and body temperature. The work of Feldberg and his colleagues [280] has shown that when 5-HT is injected into the cerebral ventricle of cats or dogs or monkeys, there follows a rise of body temperature. A similar injection in the rabbit or the sheep causes a slight lowering of temperature, but in goats or oxen there is a pronounced lowering. The action of 5-HT is in contrast to that of noradrenaline or adrenaline which, when injected into the cerebral ventricles of cats, dogs and monkeys, lower body temperature. In rabbits and sheep noradrenaline and adrenaline raise body temperature, but they have no effect in goats or oxen. The rise of temperature caused by intraventricular injection of larger doses of 5-HT in cats, such as 200 μg., is often lasting and preceded by a slight initial fall. This fall is said to be due to paralysis of cells in the anterior hypothalamus which are excited by small doses.

5-HT and vagal inhibition. Evidence has been obtained that 5-HT plays a part in transmitting impulses carried in the vagus to the stomach of the guinea-pig and the mouse [Bülbring and Gershon, 281]. For these experiments the stomach was isolated together with its vagal and sympathetic supply, and was suspended in a bath so that the intra-luminal pressure in the stomach could be recorded. Stimulation of the vagus caused an increase of pressure followed by a decrease, and 5-HT had a similar double effect. Since 5-HT was without any direct action on the muscle, the conclusion was drawn that its action was on the vagal ganglia, some of which are excitatory and others inhibitory. In the presence of hyoscine, not only stimulation of the vagus, but also nicotinic drugs like DMPP, and 5-HT caused relaxation. But there was a difference between the three agents in causing relaxation. Thus pentolinium, which is a competitive blocking agent for acetylcholine, not causing depolarization, partially blocked the effect of the vagus in causing relaxation; on the other hand pentolinium entirely blocked the action of DMPP, but had no blocking action on 5-HT at all.

A nicotinic drug like DMPP, during its early depolarizing phase, stimulated inhibitory neurones transiently, and then blocked transmission in the vagal pathway and blocked the response to 5-HT. Thus nicotinic drugs, in their depolarizing phase, antagonized both transmission through the vagal ganglia and also the response to 5-HT. Later, when the action of the nicotinic drugs changed from depolarizing to competitive, the block became specific for acetylcholine receptors only, while the inhibitory response to 5-HT returned. With this return there was a partial return of the vagal inhibitory response. Thus it appeared that the vagal inhibitory ganglia received preganglionic terminations which liberated acetylcholine and also others which liberated 5-HT.

This was supported by the finding that inhibitory vagal responses were reduced by antagonists of 5-HT without reduction of responses to nicotinic compounds, just as pentolinium reduced vagal responses without affecting those to 5-HT.

The 5-HT receptors on inhibitory neurones in the stomach behaved in the same way as neural 5-HT receptors in other tissues. They were stimulated, and later blocked, by biguanides and quaternary derivatives of 5-HT. Thus the evidence described, together with other evidence, showed that 5-HT transmitted the impulse of some of the preganglionic vagal fibres terminating around ganglia which give rise to inhibitory fibres to the stomach wall. This is a complicated story.

5-HT in peristalsis. Peristalsis begins in the intestine when the intraluminal pressure rises and reaches a threshold. The threshold is lower when 5-HT is present in the intestine and is in contact with receptors in the mucosa. Thus while 5-HT has a powerful stimulating action on peristalsis when applied to the mucosa, when applied to the serosa it inhibits peristalsis. Kottegoda [282] observed that after repeated application of 5-HT to the serosa in the presence of acetylcholine, 5-HT blocked its own action, and also blocked the reciprocal response of the two muscle layers to distension. The reciprocal response refers to the mechanism which ensures that when the longitudinal muscle contracts, the circular muscle relaxes, and vice-versa.

This inhibition of the reflex response by 5-HT in the presence of acetylcholine was similar to that produced by ganglion-blocking drugs, and this may be why 5-HT inhibits peristalsis when applied to the serosa. Kottegoda suggests that 5-HT is the transmitter released from a collateral of an interneurone which excites an inhibitory impulse to the circular muscle at the moment when the main fibre of the interneurone is exciting a motor fibre to the longitudinal muscle. Thus he conceives and supports with evidence the view that 5-HT plays the same part in peristalsis as in the guinea-pig stomach. In both 5-HT is released from the terminals of a preganglionic fibre to stimulate an inhibitory ganglion cell. His diagram should be studied.

5-HT in the pineal gland. The mammalian pineal gland was shown by Lerner to contain indole when he extracted N-acetyl-5-methoxytryptamine from the ox pineal and called it melatonin. He demonstrated the action of melatonin on the melanocytes of the frog skin. Quay and Halevy [283] showed that the pineal content of 5-HT in rats nearly doubles in the second post-natal week and then continues to increase until it reaches adult concentrations of 80 to 128 ng./mg. of fresh tissue.

Bertler, Falck and Owman [284] developed a fluorescence

microscopic method for monoamines together with a fluorimetric determination of 5-HT. They found large amounts of 5-HT, partly in the parenchyma and partly in sympathetic nerves. Although the nerves were adrenergic, having their origin in the superior cervical ganglion, they were able to take up 5-HT from the parenchymal cells into their terminal portions, so that the fibres contained two amines. Approximately half the pineal 5-HT was in the parenchyma, and half within the sympathetic fibres. An injection of noradrenaline depleted the fibres of most of their content of 5-HT.

The pineal gland is not the only situation in which nerves normally containing catecholamines take up 5-HT. Lichtensteiger, Mutzner and Langsmann [285] treated mice with reserpine and nialamide (an inhibitor of monoamine oxidase) and then gave 5-hydroxy-tryptophan. They found that the median eminence showed a yellow fluorescence characteristic of 5-HT which also appeared in most of the nerve cells within the arcuate and posterior periventricular nucleus of the hypothalamus. The yellow fluorescence was found in the same place as nerve cells containing catechol amines.

Quay made the interesting observation that there is a daily variation in the amount of 5-HT in the rat pineal which reaches its peak about midday, and reaches its lowest level about midnight. There is also a daily variation in the amount of noradrenaline which is in the opposite direction.

Zweig and Axelrod [286] have demonstrated that if the formation of noradrenaline is diminished by injecting an inhibitor of tyrosine hydroxylase (namely alpha-methyl paratyrosine) then the amount of pineal 5-HT rises. This rise can be prevented by giving dopamine, which reaches the pineal gland, since the gland is outside the blood–brain barrier.

The 5-HT in platelets. Blood platelets contain 5-HT which they probably take up when passing through the capillaries of the intestinal mucosa. The taking-up of 5-HT by platelets has been studied *in vitro* by Born and Gillson [287] who found that platelets suspended in plasma can take up 5-HT against a concentration gradient as great as 1000 to 1. The 5-HT when it is taken up is bound to ATP (adenosine triphosphate). Platelets can be made to contain 2 or 3 times more 5-HT than the amounts found in the platelets of patients with carcinoid tumours. Platelets aggregate and form clumps in the presence of adenosine diphosphate. They are also caused to aggregate by adrenaline, and in human citrated plasma by 5-HT.

CHAPTER II

PROSTAGLANDINS.
TRANSMISSION TO ANTERIOR
PITUITARY GLAND

The Prostaglandins

Prostaglandin was the name which U. S. von Euler [289] gave
to a lipid which he found in human seminal plasma and which
was physiologically active in stimulating smooth muscle. Today
many different prostaglandins have been found which are closely
related compounds. Long-chain fatty acids such as linoleic acid
are essential constituents of the diet, and from linoleic acid,
arachidonic acid is formed. Prostaglandins are synthesized from
arachidonic acid.

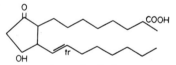

Prostaglandin E_1

Action on the reproductive tract. After coitus, prostaglandins in the seminal plasma are absorbed from the vagina in
amounts which affect smooth muscle tone and may influence
the transport of sperm in the uterus, or perhaps assist in retaining
the ovum in the Fallopian tube until it is fertilized. In the rabbit
the injection of adrenaline causes a rise in the intraluminal
pressure of the oviduct; this rise no longer occurs after the
intravenous injection of 0.4 μg. prostaglandin E_1.

Action on the blood pressure. The action of prostaglandin on the blood pressure varies with the species and also with the prostaglandin. Prostaglandin E_1 lowers the blood pressure in all species and prevents the rise of pressure caused by noradrenaline, vasopressin and angiotensin. Prostaglandin F_{2a} raises the blood pressure in the dog and the rat; this rise may be due to constriction of the veins with improved venous return to the heart, for the rise does not occur if the sympathetic fibres to the veins are cut.

Action on adipose tissue. In an anaesthetized dog a large rise in the concentration of free fatty acids in the blood follows the infusion of noradrenaline; this rise is arrested by an infusion of prostaglandin E_1, and the level of free fatty acids returns to the initial value. Again in isolated fat cells, adrenaline causes a large rise in cyclic AMP; this rise is also abolished if prostaglandin E is given together with adrenaline.

Action on the nervous system. When prostaglandin E_1, E_2 or E_3 is injected into the cerebral ventricle of an unanaesthetized cat, the condition known as catatonia develops. The cat remains in awkward positions into which its limbs are put, and takes no interest in its surroundings. When prostaglandin E_1 is injected into mice their activity diminishes and the effect of hexabarbitone in causing sleep is prolonged.

In spinal cats both prostaglandins E_1 and F_{2a} when injected intravenously cause increased tension in the gastrocnemius muscle, but this does not happen after close arterial injection. Since section of the motor nerve supply to the gastrocnemius abolishes the response, the prostaglandins must increase the firing of alpha-motoneurones, unless there is a strychnine-like action diminishing the inflow of inhibitory impulses.

Prostaglandins are released from the brain, spinal cord, spleen and diaphragm on nerve stimulation and appear to be associated with chemical transmission in some way. Ambache [290] found that antidromic stimulation of the trigeminal nerve caused miosis in the rabbit which was unaffected by atropine. The miosis was due to a lipid which he called irin. It produces vasodilatation. Recently several prostaglandins have been found in the sheep iris and irin may be a mixture of them. Irin could be concerned (Horton suggests) in antidromic vasodilatation observed elsewhere.

Control of anterior pituitary function

The Control of Ovulation. Following the coition of a male and female rabbit, central nervous reflexes are set up which lead in the female to the release of anterior pituitary hormones, and so to ovulation. The mechanism of this release is of great interest. Ovulation, however, does not depend in all species on coitus. While it does so in the rabbit and the ferret, it does not in the rat, or in the human. The rupture of a follicle and discharge of an ovum then depends on what is called the hypothalamic clock, which controls the rhythmic release of gonadotrophins. This rhythm is much affected in its timing and frequency by surrounding conditions. Thus in the human female amenorrhoea may develop in nurses on night duty, or in air hostesses who travel long distances.

One of the early steps in the investigation of ovulation was taken when it was shown that stimulation of the tuber cinereum was effective in causing ovulation.

Neurohumoral control mechanism. What has finally been demonstrated, in large part as the result of the work of G. W. Harris [294], is that the influence of impulses passing down nerves running through the hypothalamus to end in the median eminence, is not transmitted directly to the anterior pituitary, but by way of a portal system of blood vessels. This portal system starts as a plexus of capillaries in the median eminence, and then forms vessels on the pituitary stalk and finally breaks up into the sinusoids of the *pars distalis* of the pituitary gland. The anterior pituitary gland functions normally when these vessels are intact, but not when they are divided, even when the systemic blood supply is still there. The nerve endings of hypothalamic nerve tracts liberate 'releasing factors' into the plexus of capillaries, and they are carried in the portal vessels into the gland where they regulate the secretion of anterior pituitary hormones.

Thus ovarian function (taking the process in reverse) is determined by the blood concentration of anterior pituitary gonadotrophic hormones, namely the follicular-stimulating hormone, FSH, and the luteinizing hormone, LH. The secretion of FSH and LH depends on the transport of the releasing factors from hypothalamic nerve terminals by way of the portal vessels to the anterior pituitary. The releasing factors are known as FRF, which is the follicle-stimulating hormone releasing factor, and as LRF, which is the luteinizing hormone releasing factor. The hypothalamus is the centre which integrates all the influences; it has an autonomous function in maintaining anterior pituitary activity. The action of the hypothalamus is modified (1) by impulses from structures like the amygdaloid nuclei through which environmental influences are exerted, and (2) by 'hormonal feedback', that is by the concentrations of oestrogens and progestogens liberated in the blood by the ovary as a result of the action of gonadotrophins on the ovary.

Observations supporting this scheme have been made by the electron microscope which shows:

(1) that the nerve terminals in the median eminence contain synaptic vesicles as well as vesicles of neurosecretory material;

(2) that many nerve fibres end close to the vascular endothelium of primary capillaries of portal vessels in the median eminence;

(3) that there is a perivascular space with collagenous tissue between nerve terminals and endothelium;

(4) that the endothelium of the capillaries possesses fenestrations typical of those in absorptive and secretory structures.

Fluorescence methods show a high content of catecholamine, thought to be dopamine, present in the median eminence and believed to be localized in the nerve terminals impinging on the capillaries of the primary plexus of the portal vessels. (Carlsson, Falck, Hillarp and Torp [295].)

CHAPTER 12

POLYPEPTIDES INCLUDING ANGIOTENSIN

Posterior pituitary hormones. The polypeptides known for the longest time are oxytocin and vasopressin which are released from the posterior lobe of the pituitary gland. They are both octapeptides which contain a disulphide bridge. Oxytocin is formed within the cells of the paraventricular nucleus, where it exists in combination with a carrier protein, neurophysin, and from where it is transported within the axons of the cells through the stalk of the posterior lobe to the axon terminations close to the capillaries.

Vasopressin is similarly formed in the cells of the supraoptic nucleus, where it is also combined with neurophysin.

Oxytocin is released during parturition and during suckling. The rat mammary gland is so sensitive to oxytocin that it responds to any other naturally occurring substance only in a dose 1000 times as great, with the exception of acetylcholine which is blocked by atropine. It has been shown that stimulation of the sensory endings in the nipple results in an increase in the rate of electrical discharge in the paraventricular nucleus. Vasopressin is released according to the osmolarity of the blood. If the blood is dilute there is less vasopressin. It is also released after haemorrhage, and also after stimulation of the sinus nerve by carotid occlusion.

Mechanism of release. Impulses are transmitted to the supraoptic nucleus by acetylcholine but acetylcholine has no effect beyond the nucleus (see p. 106). The release from isolated rat posterior lobes can be increased by electrical stimulation or by high K$^+$; the release moreover is proportional to the calcium concentration.

Mode of action of vasopressin. Vasopressin is an antidiuretic hormone which reduces the excretion of water. It is believed to act by increasing the permeability of the distal convoluted tubules and of the collecting tubules, so that the urine comes into equilibrium with the hypertonic fluid in the renal papillae. The evidence for vasopressin increasing permeability has been accumulated from work on the toad bladder where changes in permeability are easily followed.

Angiotensin

Renin and angiotensin. Tigerstedt found that an extract of the kidney contained a pressor substance which was released after compression of the renal artery. That was in 1898. The substance was called renin and was found to be an enzyme which acted on a globulin in the plasma to produce angiotensin I, a decapeptide which is converted to a much more active octapeptide, angiotensin II, on passage through the lungs.

Release of renin in the blood. The liberation of renin follows when there is a fall of blood pressure as after severe haemorrhage, but it also occurs when there is no fall. Thus a reduction of blood volume which does not produce a fall, may lead to increased secretion of renin and formation of angiotensin. The stimulus to renin release seems to depend on the pressure in the great veins. There appears to be a reflex mechanism controlled by stretch receptors in the great veins and having its efferent component in the sympathetic nerves to the kidney.

Release of catechol amines by angiotensin. Angiotensin liberates catechol amines from the adrenal medulla, and when injected intra-arterially, 1 μg. angiotensin liberates 1 μg. adrenaline. Bradykinin has this property also, but it is about one-fifth as potent as angiotensin. Both angiotensin and bradykinin still act when the adrenals are denervated. Moreover their action in normal adrenals is not abolished by hexamethonium as that of acetylcholine is. On the other hand renin blocks the action of angiotensin and of bradykinin, but not that of acetylcholine.

Stimulation of ganglia by angiotensin. A dose of 0.1–0.3 μg. angiotensin II injected intra-arterially towards the superior cervical ganglion causes contraction of the nictitating membrane. This response is due to a stimulant action on the ganglion itself. Bradykinin has a similar but weaker action. If the injection of angiotensin is repeated, the ganglion becomes insensitive; this is unlike acetylcholine which maintains its action on repetition.

Release of aldosterone by angiotensin. When injected into the adrenal artery, renin does not cause production of aldosterone; on the other hand the injection of angiotensin does. This effect is not accompanied by release of hydrocortisone. Giving aldosterone diminishes the production of renin, just as giving hydrocortisone diminishes the release of ACTH. The secretion of aldosterone is maintained steadily during the continuous infusion of angiotensin even for several days. This is quite unlike the secretion of catechol amines which soon stops when angiotensin is infused. Probably the secretion of aldosterone is a normal function of angiotensin.

The kinins

Bradykinin. The kinins are peptides related in structure to bradykinin which is a nonapeptide. Until lately they were believed to exist only briefly in the body, being formed by the action of enzymes on a plasma globulin and then inactivated by peptidases. But bradykinin has now been found to be stored in the skin of the brown frog, and a second substance, phyllokinin, is also in an amphibian skin.

The kinin-forming system depends on a final enzyme kallikrein, which acts on kininogen to form kinin.

When the submaxillary gland is caused to secrete by stimulation of the chorda tympani nerve, there is, in addition to secretion, vasodilatation in the gland. This vasodilatation is partly due to acetylcholine, and therefore partly diminished by the injection of atropine. The remainder of the dilatation is considered to be due to kallikrein. The facts are that when the salivary gland was perfused, it was observed that during chorda stimulation kallikrein escaped into the perfusion fluid. The suggestion was therefore made that when the gland was secreting, kallikrein entered the interstitial space of the gland, and there acted upon kininogen, forming a vasodilator kinin, which caused the dilatation.

Actions of kinins. Kinins cause not only vasodilatation but also increased vascular permeability, pain and accumulation of leucocytes. Probably whenever tissues are damaged the kinin-forming system becomes active. This is known to occur in parasitic diseases [292]. Then an inflammatory response might continue as a result of continued kinin formation. Diffusion of kininogen and inactive kallikrein from blood vessels into the inflamed area might be followed by activation of the kallikrein, and so lead to more kinin formation. Some workers have evidence that leucocytes cause kinin formation and also have kininase activity. They believe that leucocytes play an important part during chronic inflammation in the continued formation of kinins [293]. (For the part played by kallikrein in glandular secretion, see Hilton and Lewis [291].)

CHAPTER 13

THE ACTION OF NICOTINE

The action of nicotine on ganglia. Nicotine was studied a good many years before acetylcholine was synthesized, and many more years before it was found in the body. Acetylcholine was shown by Dale to exert (in the presence of atropine) actions which resembled those of nicotine, and therefore he said that acetylcholine had nicotine-like actions; to-day it would perhaps be more logical to speak of nicotine as having acetylcholine-like actions.

The action of nicotine on ganglia was studied by Langley. He applied a solution of nicotine to the superior cervical ganglion of the cat, using a fine brush. He observed that the application caused a prolonged dilatation of the pupil of the eye, but that repeated application had less and less effect. He showed that when nicotine had no effect, stimulation of the preganglionic fibres was also ineffective, though stimulation of the postganglionic fibres caused a dilatation as usual. Thus he demonstrated that nicotine first stimulated and then blocked the ganglion cells so that they would no longer respond to nicotine or to preganglionic impulses.

Nicotine facilitates ganglionic transmission. An effect related to this ganglionic stimulation is that of small quantities of nicotine injected intravenously in improving the transmission across the synapse. Armitage has found that when amounts no greater than 2 μg./kg. are injected intravenously at intervals of 30 sec. for 40 min., the contraction of the nictitating membrane

H

of the cat's eye is increased by 50 per cent when the preganglionic fibres to the superior cervical ganglion are stimulated at 1/sec. The increase in the transmission produced by nicotine diminishes as the frequency of stimulation rises. Now this amount of nicotine (2 μg./kg.) is about the same as that inhaled in one puff of cigarette smoke. Thus the smoking of a cigarette which is inhaled may produce a great effect in facilitating the transmission of impulses, not only outside the brain, but also within it.

Antidiuretic action of acetylcholine. In 1945 it was shown that nicotine had an antidiuretic action [74]. This observation was made as a consequence of the discovery by Mary Pickford [75] that acetylcholine had an antidiuretic action in the dog. She produced a diuresis by giving water by stomach tube to dogs. She then injected atropine (to exclude the parasympathetic effects of acetylcholine) and then gave 1 mg. acetylcholine by intravenous injection. She observed a prompt inhibition of the diuresis, which then gradually returned as the effect of the acetylcholine disappeared. Pickford demonstrated that the effect of acetylcholine was exerted through the posterior lobe of the pituitary gland, for after removing the posterior lobe, or at least 90 per cent of it, the antidiuretic effect of acetylcholine was almost absent.

The posterior lobe of the pituitary gland is innervated by fibres from the supraoptic nucleus, and, indeed, there is evidence that the vasopressin stored in the posterior lobe may be synthesized in the supraoptic nucleus and passed along the neurohypophysial tract. In later work Pickford [76] found that she obtained an antidiuretic effect when she injected small amounts of acetylcholine directly into the supraoptic nucleus. The solution she injected contained particles of Indian ink, and by making serial sections she was able to determine where the injection had gone. Injections of saline into the nucleus were without effect. Moreover, when the pituitary gland was removed, injections of acetylcholine into the nucleus were without effect. Nicotine has the same antidiuretic action.

Nicotine in the brain. The similarity in the action of nicotine to that of acetylcholine in the body generally, so far as the effects of acetylcholine in the presence of atropine are concerned, has always been striking, and in view of the dissimilarity in chemical structure has been a challenge to the pharmacologist. In 1938 Renshaw *et al.* [265] investigated the action of carbachol (the carbaminoyl ester of choline which is not destroyed by cholinesterase) on the blood pressure of the cat, and showed that it caused a fall which was prolonged in the presence of physostigmine. They concluded that there was reason to think that carbachol acted by liberating acetylcholine from some situation where it was bound, and that much of its action was explained by this liberation. This work suggested the possibility that nicotine is a substance which like carbachol can release acetylcholine from sites where it is bound, and that the relation of nicotine to acetylcholine may be somewhat similar to the relation between tyramine and noradrenaline. So far as the action of nicotine in the brain is concerned, there is now weighty evidence to support this view.

Nicotine and the ear twitch. By preparing cats with a cannula sunk into one of the lateral ventricles of the brain (a cannula which can remain in position for months or years), Armitage and his colleagues [226, 227, 228] have studied the effect of injecting nicotine into the ventricle. In the conscious cat there are several effects following the injection of 1–100 μg., which include twitching of the ears, salivation, licking, retching and vomiting. When the injection is made into the cat anaesthetized with chloralose, the twitching of both ears can be recorded on a kymograph. In one experiment they found that the injection of 30 μg. of nicotine into the ventricle caused 11 twitches of the left ear during a period of 3 minutes without affecting the right ear. Next they injected into the ventricle 20 μg. neostigmine; this had no effect of its own and 30 min. later they repeated the injection of 30 μg. nicotine. This now produced twitching of the left ear which lasted for no less than 12 min., and caused twitching of the right ear also for 2.5 min. After the injection of neostigmine, the twitching was not only more prolonged but was also much more violent and rapid. The increase in the response to nicotine caused by neostigmine lasted for 3 hr.

That the site of action of nicotine was within the brain was evident for several reasons. When neostigmine was injected into the femoral vein, it did not increase the effect of nicotine injected into the ventricle, but physostigmine injected into the femoral vein did so. Then hexamethonium injected into the ventricle blocked the action of nicotine, but injected into the femoral vein did not. On the other hand, mecamylamine blocked the action of nicotine whether injected into the ventricle or into the femoral vein. Both physostigmine and mecamylamine are tertiary amines capable of passing the blood–brain barrier. On the other hand, both neostigmine and hexamethonium are quaternary compounds which cannot pass the blood–brain barrier. Thus they affected the action of nicotine only when they were injected so as to be within the barrier.

Effect of nicotine on the blood pressure. A further observation of great interest was that nicotine injected into the ventricle caused a fall of blood pressure. This effect was in complete contrast to the effect on the blood pressure when injected into the femoral vein and also when inhaled into the lungs, for then nicotine causes a rise of blood pressure. The fall of blood pressure produced when nicotine was injected into the ventricle was still observed after section of the vagi, and also after the injection of hyoscine. Moreover the fall was greater when the injection into the ventricle was made after the injection of physostigmine or neostigmine, so that nicotine in causing the fall of blood pressure was again acting by releasing acetylcholine. The site of action was localized in the ventral brain stem, the region from which nicotine, when injected into the ventricle, also elicits salivation and respiratory changes.

Effect of nicotine on acetylcholine formation. In 1953 F. C. MacIntosh showed that if a small tube (about 1 cm. diameter) with open ends was placed with one end firmly on the surface of the brain, fluid exuded into the tube from the brain and in the fluid acetylcholine could be found. Thus acetylcholine is constantly being formed in the brain, and its formation is increased by brain activity. For example the brain of an anaesthetized cat can be cut off from the rest of the body, leaving the eye connected by its nerves to the brain. When a light is shone in the eye, nervous impulses travel from the retina to the visual area of the cerebral cortex. When a cup is sunk into the brain surface in this area, even when no light is shone in the eye, some acetylcholine collects in the cup. But J. F. Mitchell has found that when a light is shone, the amount is greatly increased.

Armitage and Hall have found that the injection of nicotine into the ventricle of the brain causes an increased amount of acetylcholine to be released into a cup placed on the left parietal cortex of the brain. The release of acetylcholine may then become twice as great as before, or, on the other hand, if the release of acetylcholine is high already, the injection of nicotine may depress it.

Effect of nicotine on the electrocorticogram. If a cat is anaesthetized with ether, the surface of its brain can be exposed so that electrodes can be applied and the spinal cord can be divided at the 1st cervical vertebra. This division cuts out most of the sensory impulses. The cat is kept in a quiet room where there is not much light. If the ether is removed after an hour or two the cat sleeps naturally and the electrocorticogram shows waves of large amplitude and of low frequency. When a small dose of nicotine is injected into the femoral vein in the amount of 2 μg./kg., changes characteristic of arousal begin to be seen in the waves. Their frequency increases and their amplitude declines, and after about five injections the cat itself wakes up and looks around. When the injections cease the cat soon sleeps again and the waves resume high amplitude and low frequency. The same effect in the sleeping cat is obtained by introducing cigarette smoke into the air which is pumped into the trachea in the course of artificial respiration, and again about the same amount of nicotine causes arousal.

Effect of nicotine on behaviour. Remarkable effects in reinforcing effort have been obtained in rats. The rats are first kept without water for 20 hours to make them thirsty, and are then put in a Skinner box, where at one side there is a lever, and near it a hole. The thirsty rats are then trained to press the lever which raises a cup outside the hole. The rat learns that when it hears the noise of the cup being raised it can put its head through the hole and drink a small amount of water. In the course of a week or two, the rats when put in the box go at once to the lever and begin pressing. Such rats when trained press the lever from 400 to 600 times in 90 minutes. Each press is recorded electrically.

Rats so trained have had a polythene tube inserted under anaesthesia in the jugular vein. This tube is connected to a small pump at the top of the box and does not interfere with the movements of the rat in the cage after the anaesthesia is finished.

The rats were then tested on three successive days. An example may be given from one rat out of twenty in which observations were made. On the first day when saline only was pumped into the jugular vein, the rat pressed the lever 450 times in 90 minutes. On the second day when nicotine was present in the solution, so that the rat received 2 μg./kg. every 30 sec. for 20 min., the rat pressed the lever 1300 times in 90 min. On the third day when the rat received saline only, it pressed the lever 600 times in 90 min. Thus the nicotine given in amounts equivalent to those obtained by a man smoking a cigarette, doubled the rate at which the rat pressed the lever [306]. This evidence is in favour of the view that nicotine can increase the power of concentration and the determination to reach an objective.

CHAPTER 14

ACTION OF ACETYLCHOLINE ON SYM-
PATHETIC POSTGANGLIONIC FIBRES

IN 1935 v. Brücke [101] showed that acetylcholine injected into
the skin released the adrenergic transmitter from the sympathetic
fibres which cause erection of the hairs in the cat's tail. He
demonstrated that acetylcholine did not act directly in causing
erection, because he showed that the effect was blocked by
ergotamine. Later, when it was known that the transmitter was
noradrenaline, it was shown that the action of acetylcholine was
much diminished in cats which had received reserpine to remove
the noradrenaline [78]. Middleton et al. [141] showed that when
they treated a rabbit heart, which was isolated and perfused,
with atropine then acetylcholine injected into the heart was not
inactive, as might have been expected, but caused an increase in
the rate and force of the beat and also liberated an adrenaline-like
substance into the fluid leaving the heart. The fluid leaving the
heart was tested on the rectal caecum of the chicken, the rabbit
intestine and on the frog heart. The perfusate had an effect like
that of adrenaline on all three tissues, and the substance present
was later shown to be noradrenaline [232]. Acetylcholine did not
liberate noradrenaline from a heart treated with reserpine [67].

Acetylcholine has been shown to release noradrenaline from
the sympathetic fibres in the spleen [87], from the fibres to the
vessels of the rabbit ear [77], and from the fibres to the pilomotor
muscles of the cat's tail [78].

These observations might have been held to indicate the function of the acetylcholine released by sympathetic stimulation as

being to release noradrenaline in its turn. However, Ferry [130] put forward a different view. He showed that when acetylcholine was injected into the splenic artery of the cat it caused antidromic impulses to pass up the C fibres of the splenic nerve. He therefore presumed that it would also cause impulses to pass into the spleen. Thus he suggested that acetylcholine caused release of noradrenaline by first stimulating the postganglionic fibres, which in their turn released noradrenaline. Similar observations have been made by injecting acetylcholine into the left auricle of the cat heart [233].

Evidence against this conclusion has been obtained by Hertting and Widhalm [161] who injected labelled noradrenaline into cats, and then perfused the spleen. They observed the release of labelled noradrenaline after (a) stimulation of the splenic nerves, and (b) injection of acetylcholine. The release by nerve stimulation was blocked by bretylium in concentrations from 2×10^{-6} g./ml. to 10^{-5} g./ml. The release by acetylcholine was blocked only by a concentration of bretylium of 5×10^{-5} g./ml. Wolner [194] found a similar situation when he perfused the tail of the cat. Stimulation of sympathetic postganglionic fibres caused erection of the hairs, and so did injection of acetylcholine. When bretylium was added to the perfusing fluid the effect of sympathetic stimulation was blocked long before the effect of acetylcholine. Fischer, Weise, and Kopin [234] also worked on the perfused cat spleen and found that when bretylium blocked the effect of stimulation in releasing noradrenaline it did not block the effect of acetylcholine.

Despite the evidence of these three studies the suggestion has been made that Ferry's view may still be right. If the action of bretylium is that of a local anaesthetic it might block the nerve fibres at points of branching before blocking the terminations themselves. However Exley [98] studied the action of xylocholine, which was the precursor of bretylium. He compared xylocholine with the otherwise identical compound in which the methyl groups attached to the nitrogen were replaced by ethyl groups. Xylocholine and the 'ethyl' compound were equiactive as local anaesthetics, but the 'ethyl' compound was devoid of action as an adrenergic blocking agent. It has also been shown [236] that the action of the blocking agents bretylium and guanethidine is abolished by raising the concentration of calcium ions; if, however, procaine is used as a blocking agent, its action even when the concentration of procaine is as high as 1.2×10^{-4} g./ml. is not diminished by raising the calcium concentration.

Haeusler et al. [288] examined the effect of acetylcholine (and also of DMPP) on the antidromic discharge produced in the sympathetic postganglionic fibres running to the perfused heart of the cat, measuring at the same time the amount of noradrenaline released in the effluent. The infusion of acetylcholine at a concentration of 5×10^{-5} g./ml. induced asynchronous firing for the whole period of infusion (1 min.) and an average liberation of 44 ng./min. noradrenaline. Increasing the concentration of acetylcholine, or adding atropine to the perfusion fluid, restricted the antidromic discharge to a few seconds, but greatly increased the output of noradrenaline (e.g. to 346 ng./min.). Thus the electrical activity induced by acetylcholine in the nerve, which was measured by integration, was entirely unrelated to the amount of noradrenaline released. The authors found also that tetrodotoxin (1×10^{-8} M) abolished the asynchronous discharge evoked by acetylcholine, but did not appreciably influence the release of noradrenaline caused by acetylcholine.

The effect of atropine in increasing the action of acetylcholine in releasing noradrenaline can be explained by the block of the vagal receptors, so that the amount of acetylcholine free to liberate noradrenaline was much greater in the presence of atropine. A large part of the acetylcholine was not destroyed in acting on the vagal receptors.

CHAPTER 15

CALCIUM AND THE RELEASE
OF NORADRENALINE

The perfused adrenal gland. Impulses passing down the splanchnic nerve release acetylcholine which discharges the catechol amines adrenaline and noradrenaline from the adrenal medulla. Douglas and Rubin [169, 170] have studied the part played by calcium ions in this release. They have perfused the adrenal gland of the cat with Locke's solution, injecting acetylcholine into the fluid entering the gland, and collecting the fluid leaving the gland in order to measure the catechol amines contained in it. They have found that the amount of catechol amines released by a given amount of acetylcholine depends on the concentration of Ca^{++} in the perfusing fluid, being greater when the Ca^{++} concentration is greater. The release of catechol amines is not dependent on any other ion, for the release occurs when the perfusing fluid contains only sucrose, dextrose and calcium.

When the adrenal gland is perfused with Locke's solution containing the normal amount of Ca^{++}, which is 2·2 mM, then the addition of more Ca^{++} does not lead to release of catechol amines. However, when the perfusing fluid also contains acetylcholine, so that catechol amines are being released, the addition of more Ca^{++} to the perfusing fluid increases the amount of catechol amines which are released. These and other observations have been interpreted to mean that the function of acetylcholine released by the splanchnic nerves is to increase the permeability of the chromaffin cell to calcium so that calcium can enter the cell, and having done so, then the calcium releases catechol amines from their binding sites.

If the adrenal gland is perfused with Locke's solution which is Ca^{++}-free, then provided a period of 20 minutes is allowed, perfusion with Locke's solution containing a normal amount of Ca^{++} causes a release of catechol amines. This result has received the following interpretation. Under normal circumstances with an external Ca^{++} concentration of about 2 mM, the chromaffin cell membrane remains impermeable to Ca^{++}, so that a rise in external Ca^{++} does not affect the chromaffin cell. This impermeability is due to Ca^{++} which is bound in the chromaffin cell membrane. However, when the external Ca^{++} concentration is reduced to zero, the Ca^{++} which is bound in the chromaffin cell membrane is set free, and as a result at the end of 20 minutes the chromaffin cell membrane becomes freely permeable to Ca^{++}. If at this point Ca^{++} is added to the extracellular fluid to restore the normal concentration, then some of the Ca^{++} passes through the permeable membrane into the chromaffin cell and releases catechol amines.

The last observation concerning the adrenal gland which need be mentioned is that the effect of a raised amount of Ca^{++} in increasing the release of catechol amines by acetylcholine is antagonized by Mg^{++}.

The postganglionic sympathetic fibre. Ca^{++} has been found to play a role in the release of noradrenaline from the sympathetic postganglionic fibre which closely resembles that which it plays in the release of catechol amines from the adrenal medulla. Burn and Gibbons [171] used the isolated rabbit ileum, stimulating the sympathetic postganglionic fibres running with the arteries in the mesentery and observing inhibition. The size of the inhibition was seen to depend on the Ca^{++} concentration in the bath, the inhibition being greater when the Ca^{++} concentration was higher. The inhibition was reduced by the addition of Mg^{++}.

When stimulation was applied for a period of 15 minutes in the presence of a low concentration of Ca^{++}, a partial inhibition was maintained. When the Ca^{++} concentration was raised during the stimulation, the inhibition at once increased and the increase persisted until the stimulation stopped.

Observations with acetylcholine were made in the isolated atria. In the presence of hyoscine, acetylcholine does not cause inhibition, but as shown by Kottegoda [164] it increases the rate and force of the atrial beat. A similar increase in the presence of hyoscine is caused by nicotine, and it has been shown that this increase is not observed in atria taken from rabbits treated with reserpine [172]. Hence the increase is due to the release of noradrenaline. Since Goodall [173] showed that the noradrenaline in the heart disappeared after degeneration of the sympathetic nerves, it follows that the noradrenaline is present in the postganglionic fibres, and the increased rate caused by acetylcholine and by nicotine in the presence of hyoscine is due to the release of noradrenaline from these fibres. The observation was made that the increase in rate caused by acetylcholine and by nicotine was dependent on the Ca^{++} concentration in the bath, and that the increase was greater as the Ca^{++} concentration rose. The action of tyramine and of noradrenaline was not increased by a

TABLE 15.1

Effect of Ca^{++} concentration on the mean increase in rate of isolated atria in the presence of hyoscine 10^{-6}

Drug	Concentration g./ml.	Ca^{++} concentration (mM)			
		2·2	4·4	6·6	13·2
		%	%	%	%
ACh	5×10^{-5}	− 3		+19	+46
Nicotine	2×10^{-6}	+35	+100		
Tyramine	2×10^{-6}	+45		+51	
Noradrenaline	2×10^{-6}–10^{-5}	+71		+75	+33

rise in Ca^{++} concentration. The mean effects for the four substances are shown in Table 15.1.

When Ca^{++} was removed from the bath containing the rabbit ileum, the pendular rhythm usually died away in 2 minutes, and when Ca^{++} was restored at that point, the pendular rhythm was at once resumed. If, however, Ca^{++} was removed for 20 minutes, then when it was restored at the end of this time, there was little or no resumption of rhythm for a minute, and then a small rhythm began which slowly increased until it reached its previous amplitude in 3·5 or 4 minutes. Such a delay in the resumption of the rhythm might have been due to the release of noradrenaline. It was possible that as in the adrenal medulla, a period of 20 minutes without Ca^{++} might have led to a removal of Ca^{++} from binding sites in the postganglionic fibre membrane, so that the membrane then became permeable to Ca^{++}. When the Ca^{++} was replaced in the bath, it might then enter the fibre now permeable to Ca^{++}, and release noradrenaline. If in fact the delay in resumption of rhythm on readmitting Ca^{++} after 20 minutes was to be explained in this way, then the delay in the resumption should not occur if the ileum was taken from a rabbit previously injected with reserpine so as to remove the noradrenaline. Experiments were therefore carried out in rabbits treated with reserpine, and it was found that there was little or no delay in the resumption of the pendular rhythm when Ca^{++} was readmitted after a period of 20 minutes in which Ca^{++} was absent. This result rested on a comparison of the responses in the ileum of 4 normal rabbits with the responses of the ileum of 4 rabbits treated with reserpine.

These results showed that the situation in the sympathetic postganglionic fibre was very similar to the situation in the adrenal medulla. In the postganglionic fibre acetylcholine was found to release noradrenaline, this release being dependent on the external Ca^{++} concentration; in the adrenal gland acetylcholine released catechol amines, and this release was also dependent on the external Ca^{++} concentration. In both the postganglionic fibre and in the adrenal medulla a period of absence of Ca^{++} lasting 20 minutes produced a condition in which readmission of Ca^{++} caused a release of noradrenaline from the postganglionic fibre and a release of catechol amines from the adrenal medulla.

CHAPTER 16

RELEASE OF ACETYLCHOLINE BY THE SYMPATHETIC POSTGANGLIONIC FIBRES

Demonstration of fibres liberating acetylcholine. In 1934 Dale and Feldberg [14] showed that the postganglionic fibres to the sweat glands of the cat's foot transmitted their impulses by the release of acetylcholine. At this time Dale proposed that the words 'adrenergic' and 'cholinergic' should be used to 'distinguish between chemical function and anatomical origin'. 'We can then say that postganglionic parasympathetic fibres are predominantly, and perhaps entirely, cholinergic, and that postganglionic sympathetic fibres are predominantly, though not not entirely, adrenergic.'

These terms have come into general use, but those using them have not considered the problem of how noradrenaline is released. Feldberg and Minz [9] made the surprising discovery that splanchnic nerves did not release adrenaline from the adrenal glands directly and found that acetylcholine provided a cholinergic link in the transmission.

There has long been general agreement that the cells of the adrenal medulla are derived from the embryonic sympathetic nervous system. At an early stage the intra-adrenal cells are very similar to those in the sympathetic ganglia. By the 30 mm. crown-rump length stage in the human embryo some of the cells differentiate toward the structure of chromaffin cells, but for some time most of the cells have the general appearance of sympathetic neuroblasts [Boyd, 235].

Therefore, after the surprising demonstration of Feldberg and Minz, it might well have been asked whether there was another surprise in store, and whether acetylcholine was involved in the release of sympathin from the sympathetic postganglionic fibre. But no one asked this question at that time.

Evidence of release of acetylcholine by sympathetic nerves. Yet in 1931 Euler and Gaddum had made the discovery that sympathetic fibres released not only an adrenaline-like substance but also acetylcholine. Their finding arose from an investigation of the Rogowicz phenomenon, first described in 1885. This was a curious contraction of the denervated facial muscles of the dog which occurred when the cervical sympathetic nerve was stimulated. Euler and Gaddum showed that the contraction was due to the release of acetylcholine from the terminations of the postganglionic fibres coming from the superior cervical ganglion. Thus Euler and Gaddum established that fibres exerting their main effect by liberating what we now know to be noradrenaline also liberated acetylcholine.

This rather obscure phenomenon was generally forgotten when Dale and Feldberg in 1934 showed that the postganglionic fibres to the sweat glands of the cat's foot transmitted their impulses by acetylcholine alone. Since that time physiologists have paid little or no attention to evidence of acetylcholine release when this has been demonstrated in sympathetic fibres mainly concerned in the release of noradrenaline.

There were, however, by 1948 already several cases in which both noradrenaline and acetylcholine had been shown to be released by stimulation of sympathetic fibres. Thus Bülbring and Burn [71] found that both substances were released by the postganglionic fibres running to the vessels of the dog's hind leg. They showed that when the hind leg was perfused stimulation caused acetylcholine to appear in the venous effluent. In the same year Sherif [80] found that acetylcholine was released by the sympathetic fibres to the dog uterus. In 1948 Folkow and Uvnäs [83] found that both substances were released by the sympathetic fibres to the vessels of the cat's hind leg. The discovery that both substances were released by fibres innervating blood vessels was not very surprising, because it seemed reasonable that vessels should have an innervation which could cause vasodilatation as well as vasoconstriction.

Release of acetylcholine by sympathetic nerves to the heart. However, there was no such explanation for a second discovery made by Folkow, Frost, Haeger, and Uvnäs [82]. They showed that when the heart of the cat or of the dog was perfused, stimulation of the stellate ganglion led to the appearance of acetylcholine in the fluid leaving the heart. The fibres carrying the impulses are the nervi accelerantes, and their function is to make the heart beat faster and more powerfully, which they accomplish by liberating noradrenaline. What, then, could be the purpose of the release of acetylcholine?

At this point it can be said that there is no doubt that the finding of Folkow and Uvnäs and their colleagues was correct. The release of acetylcholine has been confirmed three times. First by Huković [91], who prepared the atria of the rabbit heart with sympathetic fibres attached. He set up the preparation in an isolated organ bath and stimulated the stellate ganglion; he observed an increase in the rate and force of the beat. He then injected rabbits with reserpine, and so was able to remove all noradrenaline from the sympathetic postganglionic fibres. When he prepared the atria from these rabbits he found that stimulation of the stellate ganglion caused inhibition; he found that the inhibition was greater in the presence of physostigmine, and that it was abolished by atropine. Thus stimulation caused liberation of acetylcholine.

Other experiments were carried out by Day and Rand [96] on the isolated atria of the cat; they used guanethidine to prevent the release of noradrenaline, and found that stimulation of the stellate ganglion no longer caused a simple increase in force and rate, but that the response gradually changed to inhibition. Thus before the addition of guanethidine, stimulation increased the atrial rate from 78 to 108 beats per minute, but after the addition of guanethidine [5 μg./ml.] the same stimulation decreased the rate from 84 to 56 beats per minute. Again, Boura and Green [99], working on the cat anaesthetized with chloralose, found that if they prevented the release of noradrenaline by injecting bretylium, then stimulation of the inferior cardiac nerve caused slowing of the heart instead of acceleration, and that the slowing was blocked by atropine. The combined effect of the four pieces of evidence is to establish that acetylcholine is released when the accelerator nerves to the heart of the dog, the cat, and the rabbit are stimulated, though under normal circumstances this acetylcholine exerts no effect on the heart rate.

Release of acetylcholine from the splenic nerves. Further investigation has revealed that the sympathetic nerves to the spleen resemble those to the heart in releasing both noradrenaline and acetylcholine. Burn and Rand [88] studied the response to stimulation of the splenic nerves in cats given reserpine previously to remove noradrenaline from the nerves. Stimulation did not evoke the usual response of contraction of the spleen, but on the contrary made the spleen dilate. This dilatation was shown to be due to the release of acetylcholine, because the dilatation increased after the injection of physostigmine and was abolished by the injection of atropine. More important, however, was the work of Brandon and Rand [86], who perfused the spleens of cats which had been treated with reserpine. The postganglionic fibres of these cats contained little or no noradrenaline, and when they were stimulated (neostigmine being present in the perfusion fluid) Brandon and Rand found that acetylcholine was liberated in the venous effluent.

Amount of acetylcholine in splenic nerves. These workers also measured the amount of acetylcholine and of noradrenaline in the nerves. They did this very ingeniously by following the method of Euler and Purkhold [42], who estimated the noradrenaline in the splenic nerves of sheep by determining the amount in the normal spleen and the amount in the spleen after section and degeneration of the splenic nerves. Brandon and Rand made their experiments in cats. In the normal cat spleen the amount of noradrenaline was $1\cdot13\,\mu g./g.$ and the amount of acetylcholine was $0\cdot47\,\mu g./g.$ In spleens to which the sympathetic fibres had degenerated the amount of noradrenaline declined to $0\cdot21\,\mu g./g.$ (18 per cent of the amount in normal spleens) and the amount of acetylcholine declined to $0\cdot1\,\mu g./g.$ (22 per cent of the amount in normal spleens). Since there was almost the same percentage drop for the two substances, the conclusion was drawn that about 80 per cent of the acetylcholine and 80 per cent of the noradrenaline in normal spleens were present in the nerves, and that the amount of acetylcholine in the nerves was as high as 40 per cent of the noradrenaline. Any impression that the amount of acetylcholine in postganglionic fibres is negligible must therefore be abandoned.

Sympathetic fibres to the skin of the rabbit ear. The effect of sympathetic stimulation on the vessels of the skin has always been recorded as constrictor, even when the stimulation was applied to centres in the brain and was followed by dilatation in the muscles [89]. This has led to the belief that there were no cholinergic fibres to the skin. Recently observations have been made in which stimulation was applied to the postganglionic fibres supplying the vessels of the rabbit ear. The first experiments were carried out by perfusing the vessels with a modified Ringer's solution containing eserine. The solution which issued from the vein was tested on the isolated muscle of the leech suspended in eserinized frog Ringer. The perfusate leaving the ear when the sympathetic nerves were not stimulated had no effect on the leech muscle, but that collected during stimulation caused the leech muscle to contract. This indicated the release of acetylcholine during stimulation.

A study of the changes in the vessels of the rabbit ear was also made by Holton and Rand [90] who recorded the blood flow in an area of the ear through which a source of light illuminated a photo-electric cell. Constriction of the vessels in the area led to the passage of more light through the thickness of the ear, and dilatation of the vessels led to the passage of less light. Stimulation of the postganglionic sympathetic nerves produced constriction followed by dilatation. The dilatation was increased by eserine and decreased by atropine. Guanethidine, a substance which prevents the release of noradrenaline, abolished the vaso-constriction but not the dilatation. After the superior cervical ganglion had been decentralized by degeneration of the pre-ganglionic sympathetic nerves, the vessels were more sensitive to acetylcholine and the vasodilatation in response to sympathetic stimulation was enhanced. The conclusion was drawn that sympathetic stimulation resulted in the liberation of acetylcholine which caused the vasodilatation, and that cholinergic fibres were present in the sympathetic supply to the skin vessels.

Cholinergic fibres to the nictitating membrane. The presence of cholinergic fibres to the nictitating membrane was first indicated by the experiments of Ambache [135] who found that when he injected botulinum toxin into the membrane of cats, the contraction in response to postganglionic stimulation of the treated side was reduced to a mean of 50 per cent of the contraction on the normal side. He concluded that the diminution was due to the block of the release of acetylcholine from cholinergic fibres.

The second reason for deducing the presence of cholinergic fibres was that when the head of the cat was perfused with

Locke's solution, the contractions of the membrane being recorded in response to postganglionic stimulation, addition of eserine to the perfusion fluid caused a large increase in the size of the contractions. When atropine was injected into the perfusion fluid the contractions returned to their initial size [113].

Pilomotor muscles of cat's tail. Stimulation of sympathetic postganglionic fibres has been shown to release acetylcholine into the venous effluent during perfusion of the pilomotor muscles of the cat's tail [194].

TABLE 16.1.

Stimulation of sympathetic fibres to the following tissues or organs has been shown to release acetylcholine as well as noradrenaline.

1. Buccal mucous membrane of dog [8]
2. Hind leg vessels of dog [71]
3. Uterus of dog [80]
4. Hind leg vessels of cat [83]
5. Heart of dog [82]
6. Heart of cat [82, 96, 99]
7. Heart of rabbit [94]
8. Spleen of cat [88, 86]
9. Skin vessels of rabbit ear [88, 90]
10. Pilomotor muscles of cat's tail [194]
11. Nictitating membrane of cat [88, 113]

The effect of frequency of stimulation. In the observations described, evidence has been given that stimulation of sympathetic postganglionic fibres releases acetylcholine as well as noradrenaline. How is this release of acetylcholine affected by the frequency of stimulation? An answer to this was given by observations on the nictitating membrane of the cat when contractions were evoked by postganglionic stimulation. The cats were anaesthetized with chloralose, and a series of contrac-

TABLE 16.2.

Height of contractions (mm.) of nictitating membrane in response to stimulation of postganglionic fibres by 200 shocks before and after the injection of hyoscine, 0·1 mg./kg.
(Burn, Dromey and Large, 148)

Frequency shocks/sec.	Experiment 1			Experiment 2			Experiment 3		
	Control	Hyoscine	% less	Control	Hyoscine	% less	Control	Hyoscine	% less
0·5	26	20	23	—	—	—	7	1·5	78·5
1·5	36·5	30·5	16	33	28	15	16	11	31
5·0	41	37	10	43	38·5	10·5	27	27	0
10	42	40	5	50	48	4	33	33	0
20	44	44	0	52	50·5	3	—	—	—

tions in response to a fixed number of maximal shocks applied at different frequencies was recorded. In Table 16.2 are shown the results in 3 experiments which were typical of those seen in 5 other experiments. The control observations of exp. 1 show that a frequency of 0·5/sec. caused a contraction of 26 mm., while a frequency of 20/sec. caused a contraction of 44 mm. Since these contractions were produced as a result of the release of both noradrenaline and acetylcholine, hyoscine (0·1 mg./kg.) was injected in order to abolish the effect of acetylcholine. The series of stimulations was then repeated to determine the effect of the noradrenaline alone. At a frequency of 0·5/sec. the contraction of 26 mm. was reduced by hyoscine to 20 mm., while at a frequency of 20/sec. the control contraction was not reduced at all. In each experiment the effect of hyoscine diminished as the frequency rose, indicating that the amount of acetylcholine liberated to act directly on the end organ diminished as the frequency rose.

CHAPTER 17

EVIDENCE THAT ACETYLCHOLINE LIBERATED BY SYMPATHETIC STIMULATION RELEASES NORADRENALINE

THE evidence given in the last chapter shows that sympathetic postganglionic nerves, such as those which supply the spleen and the heart, release not only noradrenaline but also acetylcholine. The possibility thus arises that the main function of the acetylcholine is to act as a link in the release of noradrenaline as in the adrenal medulla.

The perfused mesenteric arteries. McGregor [296] has described a method of perfusing the branches of the superior mesenteric artery of the rat through a cannula tied in the main artery. Tyrode solution at pH 7.4 is driven into the cannula by a pump, and emerges from the arterial branches which are cut off from the intestine, so that the tissue perfused is entirely arterial. The pump is adjusted to deliver fluid at a rate of 25 ml. per min. and the pressure in the cannula is recorded by a mercury manometer. The sympathetic fibres from the ganglion which run on the surface of the artery are stimulated by platinum electrodes using the frequencies shown by Folkow [297] to be within the physiological range, that is less than 8/sec. The vasoconstriction which results from stimulation has been shown to be unaffected by hexamethonium but to be blocked by bretylium and guanethidine.

Effect of temperature. Malik [298] found that the response to stimulation was much greater at the lower temperature of

22°C than at 35°C, but that the response to an injection of noradrenaline was much less at 22°C than at 35°C. The following results were obtained at 22°C.

Effect of acetylcholine. When acetylcholine was added to the perfusion fluid in the very low concentration of 50 pg./ml., the pressure due to the vasoconstriction caused by stimulation slowly rose for 36 min. and fell again when acetylcholine was no longer present (Malik and Ling [266]). A greater effect was obtained by

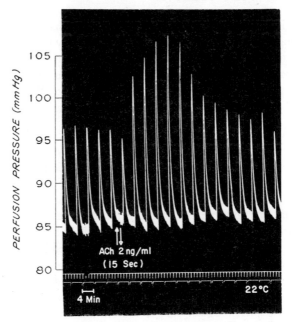

FIG. 17.1. Responses to stimulation of postganglionic fibres to the mesenteric arteries of the rat, each response showing the rise in perfusion pressure in the cannula tied in the superior mesenteric artery. When acetylcholine, 2 ng./ml., was added to the perfusion fluid for 15 sec., the response to stimulation was nearly doubled. The increase lasted for about 30 min. The stimulation was applied every 4 min. The temperature was 22°C. Maximal stimuli were given at 7/sec., duration 1 msec., for 20 sec. This and the next three figures are reproduced by permission of the Editor of *Circulation Research*.

adding acetylcholine in a concentration 40 times greater, that is 2 ng./ml. for a short period of 15 sec. This is shown in Fig. 17.1. If, however, the same concentration of acetylcholine was present in the perfusion fluid for a longer time, that is for 4 min. or more, the effect of acetylcholine was reversed, and the response to stimulation was greatly diminished. Fig. 17.2 shows this diminution when a concentration of 5 ng./ml. was allowed to act for 18 min., and it can also be seen that when the calcium

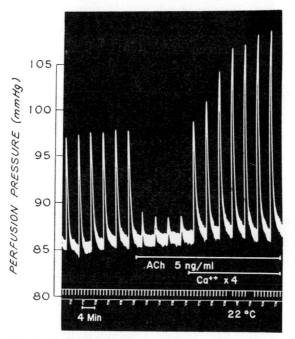

FIG. 17.2. Responses as in Fig. 17.1. A concentration of acetylcholine 5 ng./ml. was added to the perfusion fluid for 16 min. with the result that the rise of pressure due to stimulation was greatly reduced. While the addition of acetylcholine continued the calcium concentration in the perfusion fluid was increased 4-fold and then the responses to stimulation at once recovered and increased beyond their initial size.

concentration was raised, the responses to stimulation were greater than at first.

The diminution in the response to stimulation caused by acetylcholine was to some extent due to a lessening of the constrictor effect of the noradrenaline by the vasodilator action of the acetylcholine. Fig. 17.3 shows, however, that when experiments were performed in which stimulation was compared with injection of noradrenaline, acetylcholine had a much greater effect in diminishing the response to stimulation than that to noradrenaline. This was already evident when the concentration of acetylcholine was no more than 500 pg./ml. Moreover when

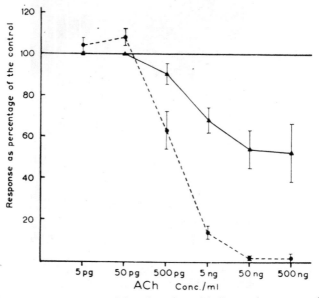

FIG. 17.3. A comparison of the effect of acetylcholine on the response of the perfused mesenteric arteries to sympathetic stimulation and to injections of noradrenaline. Solid line shows responses to noradrenaline. Dotted line shows responses to sympathetic stimulation. Each point is a mean of three experiments. The response to noradrenaline was much less affected than the response to stimulation, and was never abolished like the response to stimulation.

high concentrations were used such as 0.5 mg./ml., there was complete block of the response to stimulation which persisted long after the acetylcholine was removed, although injected noradrenaline produced a normal response.

Three further observations were made. The block produced by acetylcholine was removed by raising the calcium as is shown in Fig. 17.2, in which a fourfold rise in calcium not only abolished the block, but greatly increased the response above the height of the initial response. The block produced by acetylcholine was also reversed by d-amphetamine (0.4 μg./ml.) (Fig. 17.4). The block produced by acetylcholine was reversed by a concentration of atropine 20 times as great. Thus 0.1 μg./ml. atropine reversed the block caused by 5 ng./ml. acetylcholine [300].

Effect of DMPP. Malik and Ling [267] found that DMPP (dimethylphenyl piperazinium) in a concentration of 0.3 μg./ml.

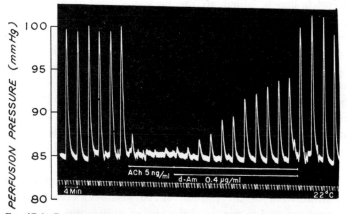

FIG. 17.4. Responses to stimulation of sympathetic fibres, and the block produced by acetylcholine 5 ng./ml. This block was reduced by adding d-amphetamine (0.4 μg./ml.). Thus the block caused by acetylcholine resembles the block produced by guanethidine.

applied for 3 min. increased the response to stimulation as did acetylcholine in a concentration of 2 ng./ml. applied for 15 sec. When the same concentration was applied for a longer time, 16–40 min., DMPP blocked the response to stimulation in the same way as acetylcholine. Moreover the block produced by DMPP was removed by raising the calcium and also by d-amphetamine. But the block was unaffected by atropine. The inclusion of guanethidine in the perfusion fluid also produced a block of the response to stimulation. This block was also removed by raising the calcium concentration and, as already shown by Day and Rand, by adding d-amphetamine. This block was unaffected by atropine.

Explanation of the double action of acetylcholine. The observations fit well with the hypothesis that when the sympathetic postganglionic fibre is excited, molecules of acetylcholine are released which act on receptors, activation of which causes liberation of noradrenaline. If a very low concentration of acetylcholine is added to the perfusion fluid at the time of stimulation, then the number of receptors activated is increased by this extra acetylcholine and the result is an increased liberation of noradrenaline as shown in Fig. 17.1. However, if the concentration of acetylcholine is allowed to act for several minutes as in Fig. 17.2, then all the acetylcholine receptors become occupied and no free receptors remain. Then the acetylcholine released from the nerve finds no receptors on which it can act, and the stimulation is without effect. Such a double effect of (1) stimulation with a little acetylcholine and (2) a block with more, is familiar at the neuromuscular junction. Thus Bülbring [302] found that the contraction of the rat diaphragm in response to stimulation of the phrenic nerve steadily increased in the presence of eserine provided the rate of stimulation was 5/min., but rapidly decreased when the rate of stimulation was 50/min. Here again too great an accumulation of acetylcholine at the higher rate reduced the number of free receptors, and so brought on block.

Thus the blocking action of acetylcholine is no indication of the presence of inhibitory receptors as Lindmar, Löffelholz and Muscholl [303] have supposed. They are motor receptors. Nor are the receptors muscarinic; they are also nicotinic. That is to say while the blocking action can be exerted by substances whose action is blocked by atropine, it can also be exerted by substances whose action is not blocked by atropine, like DMPP. Since the finding of Ambache, Perry and Robertson [268] that the superior cervical ganglion can be stimulated by muscarine, it is evident that the distinction between 'muscarinic' and 'nicotinic' has lost much of its importance. It may be nothing more than a difference of affinity. Atropine may have a greater affinity for the receptor than muscarine, and therefore blocks the action of muscarine, and so on. Just as the action of acetylcholine on the superior cervical ganglion is reduced but not abolished by atropine, so its action on the receptors at the sympathetic post-ganglionic terminals is reduced but rarely abolished by atropine depending on the relative concentrations.

Anticholinesterases. The evidence which gives the strongest support to the view that the sympathetic impulse releases noradrenaline through the action of acetylcholine was obtained from experiments in which physostigmine, neostigmine and dyflos (DFP) were used. The experiments were conducted at 30°C, since at 22°C these substances had no effect. The observations were made at frequencies from 1/sec. to 6/sec. Workers who have used higher frequencies have failed to observe an effect. Fig. 17.5 shows the result of adding neostigmine to the perfusing fluid in a concentration of 2 μg./ml. All stimulations were carried out at 1/sec. The fourth stimulus in the presence of neostigmine caused a response as great as that at 6/sec. in the absence of neostigmine. After this peak the response declined, and did so almost certainly because some block developed. This is indicated in experiments in which, while the neostigmine was present, the response diminished until it was less than the initial, and began to rise again when the neostigmine was discontinued. Fig. 17.6 shows the effect of physostigmine (6 μg./ml.) on the responses to stimulation. Physostigmine caused a slight increase in the response to noradrenaline but much less than to stimulation. Neostigmine and DFP had no effect on the response to noradrenaline. Fig. 17.7 shows the effect on the response to stimulation of DFP (2 μg./ml.) in the perfusing fluid.

Effect of higher frequencies on the increase. When stimulation was applied at higher frequencies, the increase in the response due to the anticholinesterase diminished as the frequency rose. The increase was measured as the difference between the maximum response when the anticholinesterase was present and the mean of four control responses; this difference was expressed as a percentage of the mean control response. The results are shown in Table 17.1. As the frequency rose, the time between pulses diminished and therefore the time in which cholinesterase could act was reduced. Therefore as the frequency rose cholinesterase had less effect, and therefore the anticholinesterase had less effect on the response. Table 17.1 gives the number of

TABLE 17.1.

Mean percentage increase in response

Frequency	Neostigmine 2 μg./ml.	DFP 2 μg./ml.	Physostigmine 6 μg./ml.
1/sec.	530 [10]	385 [10]	245 [10]
2/sec.	200 [8]	135 [6]	200 [6]
3/sec.	95 [6]	40 [6]	60 [6]
6/sec.	25 [6]	17 [6]	30 [7]

No. of experiments in brackets.

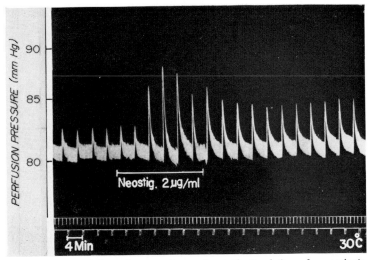

FIG. 17.5. Perfusion of mesenteric arteries, and stimulation of sympathetic fibres at a frequency of 1/sec. The temperature of the perfusion was 30°C, since at 22°C, anticholinesterases were found to have no effect. When neostigmine, 2 μg./ml., was added to the perfusion fluid, the response to stimulation at 1/sec. was greatly increased. The response remained greater than the control responses after the neostigmine was removed.

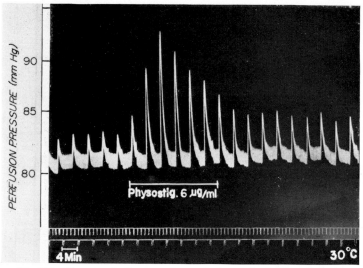

Fig. 17.6. The record of an experiment similar to the last in which physostigmine 6 μg./ml. was added to the perfusion fluid. The addition caused a large increase in the response which was not maintained because an excessive accumulation of acetylcholine led to block beginning. The fall in the response was arrested when the addition of physostigmine was stopped.

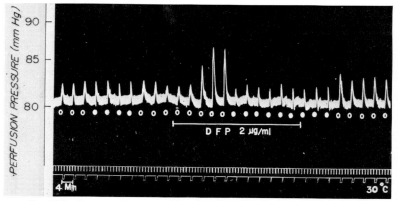

Fig. 17.7. An experiment in which the effect of DFP was tested on (1) the response to stimulation and (2) the response to injections of noradrenaline. The empty circles mark stimulations and the full circles mark injections of noradrenaline. The dose of noradrenaline was 100 ng. The addition of DFP, 2 μg./ml., increased the response to stimulation at 1/sec., but did not change the response to noradrenaline.

experiments in brackets after the percentage increase for each of the three substances at each of the four frequencies. The standard errors of the mean are not shown in the table (see 302).

Conclusions. These results, obtained from 28 to 30 experiments with each of the three anticholinesterases, provide much the clearest evidence so far that the release of noradrenaline from the sympathetic postganglionic fibre is mediated by the release of acetylcholine. Similar evidence has been obtained in seven other tissues, the cat nictitating membrane [113], the dog femoral artery [176], the taenia of the guinea-pig [198], the dog retractor penis [246], the isolated rabbit ear vessels [88], the renal blood flow in the dog [260] and the isolated rabbit heart [245]. In all of these the presence of an anticholinesterase increased the response, and in five it was shown that the increase was greatest at the lowest frequency, diminishing as the frequency rose. But in none does a superficial inspection of the records give so clear an impression as do these records from the perfused mesenteric arteries of the rat obtained by Malik [302].

CHAPTER 18

THE ADRENERGIC
BLOCKING DRUGS

Acetylcholine. The first substance which was shown to be able to block the sympathetic postganglionic fibre at its termination was acetylcholine. Von Brücke [101] observed this when studying the pilomotor muscles of the cat's tail in 1935. Acetylcholine was also shown by Burn and Rand [88] to block the vasoconstrictor fibres to the perfused vessels of the rabbit's ear. Malik and Ling [299] have shown that acetylcholine has a similar effect in the mesenteric arteries (see Fig. 17.3).

Guanethidine. The next substance to be shown to block the release of noradrenaline was closely related to acetylcholine, namely xylocholine, known as TMIO. Then came bretylium, a substance which is also an onium compound, being a derivative of dimethylethyl ammonium, and after bretylium came guanethidine. Rand and Wilson [238] have discussed the close similarity between the molecular structure of guanethidine and that of xylocholine, pointing to the conclusion that all four adrenergic blocking agents, acetylcholine, xylocholine, bretylium and guanethidine act in the same way.

Both bretylium and guanethidine resemble acetylcholine in being able in a single large dose to produce an increase in the rate of isolated rabbit auricles. Since they do not have this action on atria from rabbits treated with reserpine, it follows that the increase in rate is due to the release of noradrenaline.

The situation then is that there is a fundamental similarity between acetylcholine, bretylium and guanethidine. All three can release noradrenaline from sympathetic endings, and all three can block the release. But in the body the situation never arises in which acetylcholine, liberated by sympathetic impulses, does cause block. Acetylcholine can cause block only when it is infused in a constant stream so that it leaves no receptors free. The situation for bretylium and guanethidine is the reverse of this. When introduced into the body in a single dose, they become attached to the same receptors and, once attached, they are dislodged very slowly. Many receptors are blocked, and sympathetic tone falls. Guanethidine has the additional action of reducing the store of noradrenaline in the postganglionic endings.

Relation to calcium. The action of acetylcholine in releasing noradrenaline in isolated rabbit atria depends on the calcium concentration, the action increasing as the concentration rises (see p. 132). Equally significant is that the block of the response to sympathetic stimulation by acetylcholine, bretylium and guanethidine is diminished when the calcium concentration rises. These points suggest that the receptors on which acetylcholine, liberated by the sympathetic impulse, acts, have a similar function to the receptors on the membrane on the chromaffin cell of the adrenal medulla. When the receptors are activated, calcium enters the cell and releases the catechol amines.

The observation that when either bretylium or guanethidine has produced a block, the block can be removed by raising the external calcium, implies that a block is always relative to a particular gradient of calcium ions from outside to inside, and that the block is insufficient to prevent calcium entry if the external calcium is raised.

CHAPTER 19

BOTULINUM TOXIN,
HEMICHOLINIUM AND MORPHINE

AN important question remains whether the sympathetic impulse can release noradrenaline without the intervention of acetylcholine. The answer is given by experiments in which substances which prevent the synthesis or release of acetylcholine have been used.

Botulinum toxin. This substance has been shown to prevent the release of acetylcholine [119], and it abolishes all response to postganglionic stimulation. Ambache [135] examined the action of botulinum toxin on the sympathetic supply to the iris and to the nictitating membrane. The dual innervation of the iris made interpretation of the results difficult, but in the nictitating membrane he found that the response was always reduced by botulinum toxin, and in one of his figures it was reduced by no less than 75 per cent. The average reduction was by 51 per cent. He made his injections of botulinum toxin into the membrane itself, and by such a route it would be difficult to ensure that all postganglionic fibres were affected. He concluded that the reduction of the response was due 'at least in part to paralysis of the cholinergic fibres', but he could not exclude the possibility that the adrenergic fibres were also involved. Rand and Whaler [165] found that botulinum toxin caused block of the response of the pilomotor muscles of the cat's tail to sympathetic stimulation; the toxin was injected intradermally, experiments being done in 4 cats. The volume injected was 0.05 ml. containing 200,000 mean lethal doses (LD50), and the injection was made at the base of a tuft of hair. When 17–29 hours had elapsed, the

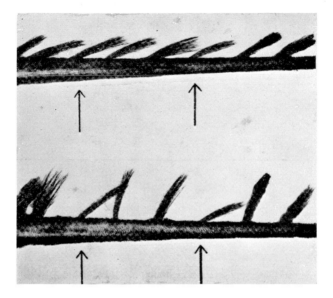

Fig. 19.1. The upper picture shows the hair tufts on the dorsal ridge of a cat's tail in their resting position. The tufts indicated by the arrows were injected at their base intradermally with 0·05 ml. botulinum toxin 18 hours previously. The tuft to the left of each arrow received 0·05 ml. of phosphate buffer. The lower picture shows the position of the tufts after 15 seconds of stimulation of the sympathetic nerves with 2 msec pulses at 10 per second. (Rand and Whaler.)

cat was anaesthetized and the sacral sympathetic trunk was stimulated. Fig. 19.1 shows that the tufts treated with toxin failed to respond while the other tufts were fully erected.

Rand and Whaler also made observations on loops of rabbit ileum set up in an isolated organ bath and stimulated through the periarterial nerves in the mesentery. Stimulation inhibited the pendular movements. When botulinum toxin was added to the bath (10,000 mean lethal doses per ml.), stimulation became completely ineffective at the end of $4\frac{1}{2}$ hours, though in a control loop of ileum the stimulation was fully effective at the end of $4\frac{1}{2}$ hours. The result was obtained in 17 out of 19 experiments.

Finally observations were made in the guinea-pig vas deferens stimulated through the hypogastric nerve. Here again botulinum toxin blocked the response to stimulation, though heat-inactivated toxin had no effect. When stimulation was blocked, noradrenaline still had its usual action in causing contraction.

Hemicholinium. The compound HC–3, one of the hemicholiniums prepared by Schueler [18], has been described in Chapter 3. It is a substance which interferes with the synthesis of acetylcholine by competing for choline, which must be transported to the site of synthesis within the neurone. Hemicholinium blocks the transport of choline, but this block is overcome by an excess of choline. In Chapter 3 the block of synthesis at the superior cervical ganglion was discussed. But hemicholinium was found to block the response of the vas deferens to stimulation of the hypogastric nerve. Since there is a ganglion on the course of the hypogastric nerve it was clear that the block might be at the ganglion rather than at the nerve termination. However, Rand and his colleagues [51, 86, 163] have shown that the response to stimulation of portganglionic fibres was blocked in the cat atria, the rabbit ear vessels, the cat spleen and the guinea-pig colon. The concentrations of HC–3 and the times to block the response are shown in Table 19.1.

In all these cases, the response was abolished and when it had been abolished it was restored with choline; the abolition was therefore shown to be due to failure of acetylcholine synthesis. It will be seen that the time taken to block was from $4\frac{1}{2}$ to $5\frac{1}{2}$ hours except for the rabbit ear vessels where it was only 3 hours. Other workers have been content to use much shorter periods and have failed to observe an effect. The molecule of HC–3 is large and can be expected to enter the postganglionic fibre only very slowly indeed.

TABLE 19.1.

Effect of hemicholinium on sympathetic postganglionic stimulation

Organ	Concentration	Time to abolition of response	Reference
Cat spleen	5×10^{-5}	263 min.	[86]
Cat atria	5×10^{-4}	270 ,,	[51]
Rabbit ear vessels	5×10^{-5}	180 ,,	[51]
Guinea-pig colon	5×10^{-5}	335 ,,	[163]

HC–3 has an action like that of hexamethonium in preventing the blocking action of bretylium [162], an action which seems to be explained by preventing bretylium from entering the postganglionic fibre. Bentley [109] also showed that HC–3 in a concentration of 10^{-4} blocked the response of the vas deferens to hypogastric stimulation within a few minutes. Since it is known that there is a ganglionic relay on the course of the hypogastric nerve, it is reasonable to suppose that HC–3 resembles hexamethonium in having a ganglion-blocking action as well. This action of HC–3 must not be confused with its specific action on acetylcholine synthesis.

The action of morphine. Morphine has been shown to reduce or abolish the response of the nictitating membrane of the cat to stimulation of the postganglionic sympathetic fibres [166]. This effect was not a depressant action on the muscle, since the direct action of noradrenaline was not reduced, and the suggestion was made that the reduction was due to a diminution in the amount of transmitter released. Morphine has also been shown to reduce the amount of acetylcholine released from cholinergic nerve endings in the guinea-pig ileum [167]. Thus morphine is a third example of a substance which diminishes the synthesis or release of acetylcholine and which also blocks the response to sympathetic postganglionic stimulation.

Comments. The failure of various workers to confirm the effect of hemicholinium in blocking the response to postganglionic stimulation has already been briefly discussed. Vincenzi and West [242] carried out experiments on an excised portion of the atria of rabbits and of cats, namely the sino-atrial node, which they stimulated, not directly through the sympathetic fibres, or through the vagal fibres, but by generalized shocks applied to the whole tissue. Stimulation caused inhibition followed by acceleration. After exposing the tissue to hemicholinium they found that the inhibition disappeared but the acceleration remained. The uncertain part of this procedure is that Blinks [262] has shown that 'the sympathomimetic effect of field stimulation is still pronounced after 2 hr. exposure to bretylium, 10^{-4} M'. He was there referring to kitten atria. He concludes that the mechanism of release by field stimulation may be quite different from that by the normal action potential. The results of Vincenzi and West are therefore ambiguous for the reason that they did not demonstrate that the acceleration which remained in the presence of hemicholinium was blocked by bretylium. This should have been done in every experiment. In the course of such work it is essential to deplete the store of acetylcholine in the sympathetic fibre, and Chang and Rand did this in their experiments by stimulating for 50 sec. every 4·5 min. Vincenzi and West stimulated only for 10 sec. every 3·3 min. The results Rand and his colleagues obtained in the cat spleen, in the rabbit ear vessels and in the guinea-pig colon, all observed during direct stimulation of the nerves, all showing abolition of the response to sympathetic stimulation, and all showing a restoration of the response by choline, give full and decisive support to the results they obtained in the intact atria.

A similar comment can be made on the paper by Vincenzi [243] in which he found that botulinum toxin failed to block the release of noradrenaline when the sino-atrial node of the rabbit was given general stimulation. He could not know how the general stimulation caused a liberation of noradrenaline, and did not discover whether it was prevented by bretylium.

CHAPTER 20

DEVELOPMENT OF THE
ADRENERGIC FIBRE

Sympathetic fibres in teleost fishes. The sympathetic post-ganglionic fibre in the mammal stands in a class by itself. The motor fibres to skeletal muscle, the parasympathetic fibres, both pre- and postganglionic, and the preganglionic sympathetic fibres transmit their impulses by releasing acetylcholine. The sympathetic postganglionic fibres to the sweat glands of the cat also transmit their impulses by releasing acetylcholine.

The other sympathetic postganglionic fibres which release noradrenaline as their main transmitter are therefore exceptional, and the question arises how they have come to differ in this fundamental respect. In the first place these sympathetic fibres do not release noradrenaline only; they release acetylcholine also. In the second place it is not true that the sympathetic fibres of all creatures release noradrenaline. Young [247] examined the splanchnic nerves supplying the intestine of two teleost fishes, *Lophius piscatorius* and *Uranoscopus scaber*. He found that the nerves were motor and not inhibitor, though adrenaline itself caused inhibition. Burnstock [248] studied another teleost fish, the trout, and obtained a similar result. He found that the splanchnic nerves were motor to the intestine, and concluded that they were cholinergic, since the response to stimulation of the nerves was blocked by atropine.

In order to see what results would be obtained in birds, a preparation of the intestine of the chicken was made similar to the preparation of the rabbit ileum described by Finkleman [261]. The periarterial nerves in the mesentery were stimulated and found to produce a powerful motor response. This response was blocked by atropine (10^{-6} g./ml.), and so appeared to be due to the release of acetylcholine. (Although sympathetic stimulation caused contraction, noradrenaline caused inhibition in concentrations from 2×10^{-8} g./ml.) While the motor response predominated in all pieces of intestine when first set up in the isolated organ bath, a small inhibition preceding the motor response was seen when the intestine had been in the bath for some hours. By this time the intestine had developed some degree of spasm, so that inhibition was more readily seen. However, this inhibition was very slight compared with that seen in rabbit intestine.

Sympathetic fibres in newborn mammals. On the view that the sympathetic fibres of the teleost fishes and of the birds have changed in the course of evolution from motor fibres to inhibitor fibres, it seemed worth while to investigate the tissues of newborn mammals to see if ontogeny recapitulated phylogeny, and whether the newborn rabbit differed from the adult rabbit. The Finkleman preparation was used again in which, in the adult rabbit, stimulation always produces inhibition. In one experiment on a rabbit 3 days old, the responses to stimulation at frequencies of 3/sec., 5/sec., 10/sec. and 20/sec. were motor, and in a second 3-day-old rabbit from another litter, the responses to frequencies of 3/sec. and 5/sec. were motor, but the responses to 10/sec. and 20/sec. were inhibitor, though the inhibition was very slight. In this experiment the addition of hyoscine (0·1 μg./ml.) to the bath abolished the motor response to stimulation at 3/sec. The response in a 12-day-old rabbit to stimulation at 50/sec. was inhibition [96], and the responses of the ileum of an 8-day-old kitten were inhibitor.

Effect of sympathetic stimulation on blood vessels. In newborn puppies Boatman, Shaffer, Dixon and Brody [249] found that when they perfused the vessels of the hind legs, stimulation of the sympathetic fibres caused vasodilatation despite the fact that the blood pressure was low, being about 30 mm. Hg. The dilatation was abolished by the intravenous injection of atropine sulphate 0·2 mg. per kg., which indicated that the dilatation was due to the release of acetylcholine. Adrenaline (2 μg.) given intra-arterially caused a rise of peripheral resistance. The decrease in vascular resistance on sympathetic stimulation was still seen not only on the first day of life, but up to 2 weeks; however, stimulation produced an increase in peripheral vascular resistance in dogs 4 weeks old and over.

Reversal of the adult response. As already described in Chapter 7 the constrictor response of the hind leg vessels of the adult dog to sympathetic stimulation can be reversed to the condition which has just been described in the newborn puppy, either by allowing the sympathetic nerve endings in the vessels to suffer from anoxia, or by treating the dog with reserpine. Sympathetic stimulation then releases acetylcholine and causes vasodilatation. By adding adrenaline or noradrenaline to the blood, the constrictor effect of stimulation can be restored, because of uptake of noradrenaline by the sympathetic nerves.

Time in which uptake occurs. Uptake occurs as the animal grows older, and the time at which it occurs has been studied in the rat heart by Glowinski et al. [255]. They found that the uptake of noradrenaline was deficient at birth, but that it increased rapidly after 8 days. In the second week after birth there was indeed a threefold increase in the capacity of the rat heart to take up noradrenaline. When there was uptake in the adult rat, what was taken up was retained, as shown by a comparison of the amount in the heart 0·5 hr. after administration with the amount present 2·5 hr. later.

In the young rat, however, up to 3 weeks old, 50 per cent of what was taken up was not retained. The retention did not reach adult levels until 6 weeks of age.

The change in the response to sympathetic stimulation in the growing animal seems to be due to the initiation of this uptake process.

Uptake of phenylalanine. Tyramine causes a rise of blood pressure by releasing noradrenaline from the sympathetic fibres. Burn and Rand [44] studied the recovery of the pressor action of tyramine in the rat previously treated with reserpine. They found that the pressor action was restored not only by infusion of noradrenaline but also by infusion of phenylalanine. Thus they showed that the precursor phenylalanine could be taken up by the sympathetic fibre, and could restore the pressor action, not for a brief interval as did the infusion of noradrenaline, but for a longer time. The development of the adrenergic fibre, absent in the first few days of mammalian life, may therefore depend entirely on the uptake process. The sympathetic fibre may take up phenylalanine from the blood and convert it to noradrenaline. The fibre which takes up phenylalanine may be a fibre which up to that time was a fibre releasing acetylcholine, but when a store of noradrenaline has been accumulated in it, the acetylcholine which was previously released to act on the end organ, now assumes the function of releasing noradrenaline.

The view can also be held that the sympathetic fibre which takes up phenylalanine and converts it to noradrenaline is not a fibre which releases acetylcholine, but is a fibre which before the uptake process began was completely inactive, and which reverts to inactivity in the adult during anoxia or after treatment with reserpine. At the present time there is no evidence which of the alternative views is correct. The release of noradrenaline has been shown to be caused by the preceding release of acetyl-choline, and if this acetylcholine comes from a different fibre from that in which the noradrenaline is held, then it follows that impulses which pass directly down fibres holding noradrenaline are ineffective, and that noradrenaline is released only by impulses passing down fibres which release acetylcholine.

CHAPTER 21

THE ANATOMICAL BASIS

THE evidence has now been described which shows that the release of noradrenaline is effected by acetylcholine. What is the anatomical arrangement? Does the acetylcholine come from a cholinergic fibre, and the noradrenaline from an adrenergic fibre? Or do both substances come from the same fibre?

The answer appears to be that both substances come from the same fibre. This answer is given by the work of Eränkö and his colleagues (*Histochemical Journal* (1970), 2, 479–489). They have studied the innervation of the rat pineal gland, which comes entirely from the superior cervical ganglion. 'Pineal glands of adult albino rats were examined histochemically using, first, formaldehyde-induced fluorescence to study mono-amines and, second, copper thiocholine or copper ferrocyanide methods to study acetylcholinesterase and non-specific cholin-esterase by light and electron microscopy. Cholinesterase was determined quantitatively by a constant pH titration assay.

Fluorescent and acetylcholinesterase-positive nerve nets formed identical patterns. Non-specific cholinesterase was observed only in nerve trunks outside the pineal. Bilateral removal of superior cervical ganglia resulted in complete dis-appearance of fluorescence and acetylcholinesterase from nerve fibres. Electron microscopically, acetylcholinesterase was found on sympathetic axons containing small granular vesicles (see Fig. 21.1). Quantitative cholinesterase determinations suggested that the pineal activity was mainly due to acetylcholinesterase. Comparison of the incubation times required for equal histochem-ical acetylcholinesterase reactions suggested that the activity of the sympathetic nerve fibres in the pineal is of the same order of magnitude as in the nerve fibres of the iris.'

The electron microscope pictures show the reaction product with thiocholine closely surrounding the axon which contains small granular vesicles. The acetylcholinesterase is thus situated between the cell membrane and the axon membrane.

Observations have also been made by Waterson, Hume and de la Lande [305] in which they have shown the presence of acetylcholinesterase and butyrylcholinesterase in transverse sections of the rabbit ear artery. The thiocholine method showed staining at the medial–adventitial border of the artery where sympathetic nerves are present. Degeneration of the sympathetic nerves following removal of the superior cervical ganglion abolished the staining, but treatment of rabbits with reserpine to remove noradrenaline did not affect the staining which was still found. These results, obtained in a situation where the sympathetic postganglionic supply is adrenergic, illustrate the finding that all fibres which liberate noradrenaline are in the closest connection with fibres supplying acetylcholine. Other examples are shown in Table 16.1.

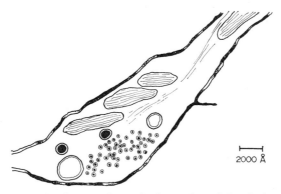

Fig. 21.1. Drawing from Eränkö, Rechardt, Eränkö and Cunningham. Distribution of acetylcholinesterase in the pineal gland. Fixation in formaldehyde-glutaraldehyde mixture. Preincubation with 10^{-5}M iso-OMPA and incubation with acetylthiocholine and 10^{-5}M iso-OMPA for 1 hour at pH 6.5. The reaction product around the axon containing small granular vesicles is situated between the axon membrane and the cell membrane. The length of the calibration line is 2000 Å.

CHAPTER 22

IMMUNO-SYMPATHECTOMY

It is possible to inject new-born animals with an extract containing antibodies which prevent the development of a part of the sympathetic system. In 1948 Bueker implanted a mouse sarcoma into chick embryo. He found that sensory fibres from the chick embryo branched into the tumour. In 1952 Levi-Montalcini showed that not only fibres from sensory ganglia but also from sympathetic ganglia were involved, and that both kinds of ganglia were enlarged, often six-fold. It was shown that the tumour released a diffusible substance which caused the ganglia to develop, and that direct contact with the tumour was not needed. The nerve growth factor was found in the microsomal fraction of the tumour, and Cohen in 1954 attempted to inactivate the nucleic acids present in this fraction by using snake venom as a source of phosphodiesterase. To his surprise he found that the snake venom itself was a rich source of the nerve growth factor, and then, since the venom comes from the salivary gland of the snake, he tested an extract from the salivary glands of the mouse and found the factor present in the male in a concentration 6000 times greater than that in tumour. The agent is a protein which is heat-labile, cannot be dialyzed, resistant to 0.1 N alkali but destroyed by 0.1 N acid. The nerve growth factor appears to be localized in the tubular portion of the salivary glands, more being present in the male than in the female, and being absent before puberty. Since it is a protein it can be injected into rabbits which then form antibodies to it. If the serum from a treated rabbit is collected, it can be used to produce a partial destruction of the sympathetic system in new-born mice and rats. This happens because the antibodies in the serum neutralize the nerve growth factor in the new-born animals, and in its absence many of the sympathetic ganglia cannot develop. In particular the ganglia of the sympathetic chain are affected, and remain minute compared with those in an untreated animal; the cell population of the ganglia is from 2 to 10 per cent of normal for mice and rats. It is therefore not surprising that the amount of noradrenaline present in organs such as the heart, the spleen and the lung is very greatly reduced, though in the brain there is no deficiency. Moreover the uptake of noradrenaline by the heart of the rat is only a small percentage of normal. In the rat iris the network of fluorescent fibres normally seen is completely lacking [Levi-Montalcini and Angeletti, 263].

An investigation carried out by Vogt [264] showed that while the superior cervical ganglion, the stellate ganglion and the ganglia of the paravertebral chain are greatly reduced by the antiserum, the coeliac and mesenteric ganglia are not obviously affected either in size or nerve cell density. This may account for the fact that gastro-intestinal function and reproduction are normal in the immuno-sympathectomized rat. Thus the antiserum is very specific, choosing some ganglia for attack, but leaving others unimpaired.

REFERENCES

[1] DALE H. H. (1914) *J. Pharmacol. exp. Ther.* **6**, 147

[2] LOEWI O. (1921) *Pflüg. Arch. ges. Physiol.* **189**, 239

[3] FÜHNER H. (1918) *Arch. exp. Path. u. Pharmak.* **82**, 51

[4] LOEWI O. and NAVRATIL E. (1926) *Pflüg. Arch. ges. Physiol.* **214**, 678 and 689

[5] DALE H. H. and GASSER H. S. (1926) *J. Pharmacol. exp. Ther.* **29**, 53

[6] DALE H. H. and DUDLEY H. W. (1929) *J. Physiol.* (Lond.) **68**, 97

[7] DALE H. H. and GADDUM J. H. (1930) *J. Physiol.* (Lond.) **70**, 109

[8] EULER U. S. v. and GADDUM J. H. (1931) *J. Physiol.* (Lond.) **73**, 54

[9] FELDBERG, W. S. and MINZ B. (1933) *Pflüg. Arch. ges. Physiol.* **233**, 567

[10] CHANG H. C. and GADDUM J. H. (1933) *J. Physiol.* (Lond.) **79**, 255

[11] FELDBERG W. and KRAYER O. (1933) *Arch. exp. Path. Pharmak.* **172**, 170

[12] KIBJAKOW A. W. (1933) *Pflüg. Arch. ges. Physiol.* **232**, 432

[13] FELDBERG W. and GADDUM J. H. (1934) *J. Physiol.* (Lond.) **81**, 305

[14] DALE H. H. and FELDBERG W. (1934) *J. Physiol.* (Lond.) **82**, 121

[15] DALE H. H., FELDBERG W. and VOGT M. (1936) *J. Physiol.* (Lond.) **86**, 353

[16] BROWN G. L., DALE H. H. and FELDBERG W. (1936) *J. Physiol.* (Lond.) **87**, 394

[17] BÜLBRING E. and BURN J. H. (1941) *J. Physiol.* (Lond.) **100**, 337

[18] SCHUELER F. W. (1955) *J. Pharmacol. exp. Ther.* **115**, 127

[19] MACINTOSH F. C., BIRKS R. I. and SASTRY P. B. (1956) *Nature* (Lond.) **178**, 1181

[20] BIRKS R. I. and MACINTOSH F. C. (1961) *Can. J. Biochem. Physiol.* **39**, 787

[21] BURN J. H. and DALE H. H. (1915) *J. Pharmacol. exp. Ther.* **6**, 417

[22] PATON W. D. M. and ZAIMIS E. J. (1948) *Nature* (Lond.) **162**, 810

[23] HARINGTON M. and ROSENHEIM M. L. (1954) *Lancet* **i**, 7

[24] FATT P. and KATZ B. (1952) *J. Physiol.* (Lond.) **117**, 109

[25] BÜLBRING E. (1946) *Brit. J. Pharmacol.* **1**, 38

[26] BOWMAN W. C. and RAND M. J. (1961) *Brit. J. Pharmacol.* **17**, 176

[27] RIKER W. F. Jr. (1953) *Pharmacol. Rev.* **5**, 1

[28] KRNJEVIĆ K. and MILEDI R. (1958) *J. Physiol.* (Lond.) **141**, 291

[29] CANNON W. B. and URIDIL J. E. (1921) *Amer. J. Physiol.* **58**, 353

[30] CANNON W. B. and BACQ Z. M. (1931) *Amer. J. Physiol.* **96**, 392

[31] EULER U. S. v. (1946) *Acta physiol. scand.* **12**, 73

[32] PEART W. S. (1949) *J. Physiol.* (Lond.) **108**, 491

[33] SCHÜMANN H. J. (1948) *Klin. Wochschr.* **26**, 204

[35] AXELSSON J., BUEDING E. and BÜLBRING E. (1961) *J. Physiol.* (Lond.) **156**, 357

[36] BUEDING E., BÜLBRING E., GERCKEN G. and KURIYAMA H. (1963) *J. Physiol.* (Lond.) **166**, 8P.

[40] HOLZBAUER M. and VOGT M. (1956) *J. Neurochem.* **1**, 8

[41] CARLSSON A. and HILLARP N. A. (1956) *K. fysiogr. Sällsk. Lund Forh.* **26**, No. 8

[42] EULER U. S. v. and PURKHOLD A. (1951) *Acta physiol. scand.* **24**, 212

[43] BURN J. H. and RAND M. J. (1958) *J. Physiol.* (Lond.) **144**, 314

[44] BURN J. H. and RAND M. J. (1960) *Brit. J. Pharmacol.* **15**, 47

[46] WHITBY L. G., AXELROD J. and WEIL-MALHERBE H. (1961) *J. Pharmacol. exp. Ther.* **132**, 193

[47] MUSCHOLL E. (1960) *Naunyn-Schmiedeberg's Arch. exp. Path. Pharmakol.* **240**, 234

[48] HERTTING G., AXELROD J., KOPIN I. J. and WHITBY L. G. (1961) *Nature* (Lond.) **189**, 66

[49] AXELROD J., WEIL-MALHERBE H. and TOMCHICK R. (1959) *J. Pharmacol. exp. Ther.* **127**, 251

[50] AXELROD J. (1957) *Science* **126**, 400

[51] CHANG V. and RAND M. J. (1960) *Brit. J. Pharmacol.* **15**, 588

[52] LINDMAR R. and MUSCHOLL E. (1961) *Naunyn-Schmiedeberg's Arch. exp. Path. Pharmakol.* **241**, 528

[53] HAGEN P. and BARRNETT R. J. (1960) *Adrenergic Mechanisms* p. 83. J. & A. CHURCHILL, London

[54] SCHÜMANN H. J. (1960) *Naunyn-Schmiedeberg's Arch. exp. Path. Pharmakol.* **238**, 41

[55] CROUT J. R., MUSKUS A. J. and TRENDELENBURG U. (1962) *Brit. J. Pharmacol.* **18**, 600

[56] BURN J. H. (1932) *J. Pharmacol. exp. Ther.* **46**, 75

[57] MELTZER S. J. (1904) *Amer. J. Physiol.* **11**, 37

[58] MACMILLAN W. H., SMITH D. J. and JACOBSON J. H. (1962) *Brit. J. Pharmacol.* **18**, 39

[59] AZARNOFF D. L. and BURN J. H. (1961) *Brit. J. Pharmacol.* **16**, 335

[61] BEJRABLAYA D., BURN J. H. and WALKER J. M. (1958) *Brit. J. Pharmacol.* **13**, 461

[62] FRÖHLICH A. and LOEWI O. (1910) *Arch. exp. Path. Pharmakol.* **62**, 160

[63] TAINTER M. L. and CHANG D. K. (1927) *J. Pharmacol. exp. Ther.* **30**, 193

[64] DE EDS F. (1927) *Proc. Soc. exp. Biol. Med.* **24**, 551

[65] TRENDELENBURG U. (1959) *J. Pharmacol. exp. Ther.* **125**, 55.

[66] MUSCHOLL E. (1961) *Brit. J. Pharmacol.* **16**, 352

[67] BURN J. H. and RAND M. J. (1958) *Brit. Med. J.* **1**, 137

[68] HUKOVIĆ S. (1959) *Brit. J. Pharmacol.* **14**, 372

[69] BURN J. H. and ROBINSON J. (1952) *Brit. J. Pharmacol.* **7**, 304

[70] BÜLBRING E. and BURN J. H. (1940) *J. Pharmacol. exp. Ther.* **68**, 150

[71] BÜLBRING E. and BURN J. H. (1935) *J. Physiol.* (Lond.) **83**, 483

[72] VAN ROSSUM J. M., VAN DER SCHOOT J. B. and HURKMANS J. A. T. M. (1962) *Experientia*, **18**, 229.

[73] AXELROD J., HERTTING G. and POTTER L. (1962) *Nature* (Lond.) **194**, 297

[74] BURN J. H., TRUELOVE L. H. and BURN I. (1945) *Brit. Med. J.* **i**, 403

[75] PICKFORD M. (1939) *J. Physiol.* (Lond.) **95**, 226.

[76] PICKFORD M. (1947) *J. Physiol.* (Lond.) **106**, 264

[77] BURN J. H. and RAND M. J. (1958) *Brit. Med. J.* **i**, 903

[78] BURN J. H., LEACH E. H., RAND M. J. and THOMPSON J. W. (1959) *J. Physiol.* (Lond.) **148**, 332

[79] GILLESPIE J. S. and MACKENNA B. R. (1960) *J. Physiol.* (Lond.) **152**, 191

[80] SHERIF M. A. F. (1935) *J. Physiol.* (Lond.) **85**, 298

[81] BACQ Z. M. and FREDERICQ H. (1935) *Arch. Int. Physiol.* **40**, 297

[82] FOLKOW B., FROST J., HAEGER K. and UVNÄS B. (1948) *Acta physiol. scand.* **15**, 421

[83] FOLKOW B., HAEGER K. and UVNÄS B. (1948) *Acta physiol. scand.* **15**, 401

[84] BÜLBRING E. and BURN J. H. (1936) *J. Physiol.* (Lond.) **87**, 254

[85] DALE H. H. (1933) *J. Physiol.* (Lond.) **80**, 10.

[86] BRANDON K. W. and RAND M. J. (1961) *J. Physiol.* (Lond.) **157**, 18

[87] DALY M. DE B. and SCOTT M. J. (1961) *J. Physiol.* (Lond.) **156**, 246

[88] BURN J. H. and RAND M. J. (1960) *Brit. J. Pharmacol.* **15**, 56

[89] LINDGREN P. and UVNÄS B. (1953) *Circulation Res.* **1**, 479

[90] HOLTON P. and RAND M. J. (1962) *Brit. J. Pharmacol.* **19**, 513

[91] HUKOVIĆ S. (1959) *Brit. J. Pharmacol.* **14**, 372

[92] GARRY R. C. and GILLESPIE J. S. (1955) *J. Physiol.* (Lond.) **128**, 557

[93] GILLESPIE J. S. and MACKENNA B. R. (1961) *J. Physiol.* (Lond.) **156,** 17

[94] HUKOVIĆ S. (1961) *Brit. J. Pharmacol.* **16,** 188

[95] EMMELIN N. and ENGSTRÖM J. (1960) *J. Physiol.* (Lond.) **153,** 1

[96] DAY M. D. and RAND M. J. (1961) *Brit. J. Pharmacol.* **17,** 245

[97] HEY P. and WILLEY G. L. (1954) *Brit. J. Pharmacol.* **9,** 471

[98] EXLEY K. A. (1957) *Brit. J. Pharmacol.* **12,** 297

[99] BOURA A. L. A. and GREEN A. F. (1959) *Brit. J. Pharmacol.* **14,** 536

[100] MAXWELL R. A., PLUMMER A. J., SCHNEIDER F., POVALSKI H. and DANIEL A. E. (1960) *J. Pharmacol. exp. Ther.* **68,** 301

[101] BRÜCKE F. (1935) *Klin. Wochschr.* **14,** 7

[102] COON J. B. and ROTHMAN S. (1940) *J. Pharmacol. exp. Ther.* **68,** 301

[106] DIXIT B. N., GULATI O. D. and GOKHALE S. D. (1961) *Brtt. J. Pharmacol.* **17,** 372

[107] BURN J. H. and FROEDE H. (1963) *Brit. J. Pharmacol.* **20,** 378

[109] BENTLEY G. A. (1962) *Brit. J. Pharmacol.* **19,** 85

[110] WILSON A. B. (1962) *J. Pharm. Pharmacol.* **14,** 700

[111] BURN J. H. and WEETMAN D. F. (1963) *Brit. J. Pharmacol.* **20,** 74

[112] FELDBERG W. and VARTIAINEN A. (1935) *J. Physiol.* (Lond.) **83,** 103

[113] BURN J. H., RAND M. J. and WIEN R. (1963) *Brit. J. Pharmacol.* **20,** 83

[114] ABRAHAMS V. C., KOELLE G. B. and SMART P. (1957) *J. Physiol.* (Lond.) **139,** 137

[115] GERSCHENFELD H. M., TRAMEZZANI J. H. and DE ROBERTIS E. (1960) *Endocrinology* **66,** 741

[116] KOELLE G. B. (1961) *Nature* (Lond.) **190,** 208

[117] PATON W. D. M. (1961) *Proc. Roy. Soc. B.* **154,** 21

[118] FATT P. and KATZ B. (1951) *J. Physiol.* (Lond.) **115,** 320

[119] BURGEN A. S. V., DICKENS F. and ZATMAN L. J. (1949) *J. Physiol.* (Lond.), **109,** 10

[120] WATLAND D. C., LONG J. P., PITTINGER C. B. and CULLEN S. C. (1957) *Anesthesiol.* **18,** 883

[121] ZAIMIS E., CANNARD T. H., PRICE H. L. (1958) *Science* **128,** 34

[122] BURN J. H. and RAND M. J. (1958) *Brit. J. Pharmacol.* **13,** 471

[123] STEPHENSON R. P. (1956) *Brit. J. Pharmacol.* **11,** 379

[124] DAY M. D. and RAND M. J. (1963) *J. Pharm. Pharmacol.* **15,** 221

[125] BURN J. H. and RAND M. J. (1960) *J. Physiol.* (Lond.) **150,** 295

[126] HERTTING G. and AXELROD J. (1961) *Nature* (Lond.) **192,** 172

[127] BURN J. H. and RAND M. J. (1959) *Brit. Med. J.,* **1,** 394

[128] WALKER J. M. (1949) *Quart. J. Med.* (N.S.) **18,** 51

[129] STEPHENSON, R. P. (1948) *J. Physiol.* (Lond.) **107,** 162

[130] FERRY C. B. (1963) *J. Physiol.* (Lond.) **167,** 487

[131] OTSUKA M. and ENDO M. (1960) *J. Pharmacol. exp. Ther.* **128,** 273

[132] HERTTING G., AXELROD J. and PATRICK R. W. (1962) *Brit. J. Pharmacol.* **18,** 161

[133] BHAGVAT B. and SHIDEMAN F. E. (1963) *Brit. J. Pharmacol.* **20,** 56

[134] COUPLAND R. E. and HEATH I. D. (1961) *J. Endocrin.* **22,** 59

[135] AMBACHE N. (1951) *J. Physiol.* (Lond.) **113,** 1

[136] BURN J. H. and RAND M. J. (1959) *Nature* (Lond.) **184,** 163

[137] BURN J. H. (1933) *Proc. Roy. Soc. Med.* **27,** 31

[138] BURN J. H. (1932) *J. Physiol.* (Lond.) **75,** 144

[139] BÜLBRING E., BURN J. H. and ELIO F. J. DE (1948) *J. Physiol.* (Lond.) **107,** 222

[140] PARKS V. J., SANDISON A. G., SKINNER S. L. and WHELAN R. F. (1961) *Clinical Sci.* **20,** 289

[141] HOFFMANN F., HOFFMANN H., MIDDLETON S. and TALESNIK J. (1945) *Amer. J. Physiol.* **144,** 189

[142] AHLQUIST R. P. (1948) *Amer. J. Physiol.* **153,** 586

[143] VAUGHAN WILLIAMS E. M. and SEKIYA A. (1963) *Lancet* **i,** 420

[144] EULER U. S. v. and LISHAJKO F. (1963) *Acta physiol. scand.* **57,** 468

[145] AXELROD J., GORDON E., HERTTING G., KOPIN I. J. and POTTER L. T. (1962) *Brit. J. Pharmacol.* **19,** 56

[147] STAFFORD A. (1963) *Brit. J. Pharmacol.* **21,** 361

[148] BURN J. H., DROMEY J. J. and LARGE B. J. (1963) *Brit. J. Pharmacol.* **21,** 97

[149] SPECTOR S., SJOERDSMA A. and UDENFRIEND S. (1965) *J. Pharmacol. exp. Ther.* **147,** 86

[151] HAMER J., GRANDJEAN T., MELENDEZ L. and SOWTON G. E. (1964) *Brit. med. J.* **ii,** 720

[152] PRICHARD B. N. C. and GILLAM P. M. S. (1964) *Brit. med. J.* **ii,** 725

[153] PAYNE J. P. and SENFIELD R. M. (1964) *Brit. med. J.* **i,** 603

[154] IVERSEN L. L. (1963) *Brit. J. Pharmacol.* **21,** 523

[155] BLACKWELL B. and MARLEY E. (1964) *Lancet* **i,** 530

[156] COOPER A. J., MAGNUS R. V. and ROSE M. J. (1964) *Lancet* **i,** 527

[157] HODGE J. V., NYE E. R., EMERSON G. W. (1964) *Lancet* **i,** 1108

[158] LINDMAR R. and MUSCHOLL E. (1964) Naunyn-Schmiedeberg's *Arch. exp. Path. Pharmakol.* **247,** 469

[159] GILLESPIE J. S. and KIRPEKAR S. M. (1965) *J. Physiol* (Lond.) **176,** 205

[160] BURGEN A. S. V. and IVERSEN L. L. (1965) *Brit. J. Pharmacol.,* **25,** 34

[161] HERTTING G. and WIDHALM S. (1965) Naunyn-Schmiedeberg's *Arch. exp. Path. u. Pharmak.* **250,** 257

[162] BURN J. H. and GIBBONS W. R. (1964) *Brit. J. Pharmacol.* **22,** 549

[163] RAND M. J. and RIDEHALGH A. (1965) *J. Pharm. Pharmacol.* **17,** 144

[164] KOTTEGODA S. R. (1953) *Brit. J. Pharmacol.* **8,** 83

[165] RAND M. J. and WHALER B. C. (1965) *Nature* (Lond.) **206,** 588

[166] TRENDELENBURG U. G. (1957) *Brit. J. Pharmacol.* **12,** 79

[167] PATON W. D. M. (1957) *Brit. J. Pharmacol.* **12,** 119

[168] BURN J. H. and SELTZER J. (1965) *J. Physiol.* (Lond.), **179,** 569

[169] DOUGLAS W. W. and RUBIN R. P. (1961) *J. Physiol.* (Lond.) **159,** 40

[170] DOUGLAS W. W. and RUBIN R. P. (1963) *J. Physiol.* (Lond.) **167,** 288

[171] BURN J. H. and GIBBONS W. R. (1964) *Brit. J. Pharmacol.* **22,** 540

[173] GOODALL McC. (1951) *Acta physiol scand.* **24,** Suppl. 85

[174] GARRY R. C. and GILLESPIE J. S. (1955) *J. Physiol.* (Lond.) **128,** 557

[175] FOLKOW B. (1955) *Physiol. Rev.* **35,** 629

[176] BERNARD P. J. and DE SCHAEPDRYVER A. F. (1964) *Arch. Internat. Pharmacodyn.* **148,** 301

[178] MUSCHOLL E. and VOGT M. (1964) *Brit. J. Pharmacol.* **22,** 193

[179] LANGLEY J. N. and ANDERSON H. K. (1895) *J. Physiol* (Lond.) **19,** 85

[181] WOLFE D. E., POTTER L. T., RICHARDSON K. C. and AXELROD J. (1962) *Science* **138,** 440

[185] RICHARDSON K. C. (1964) *Amer. J. Anat.* **114,** 173

[186] KOELLE G. B. (1963) *Pharmacology of Cholinergic and Adrenergic Transmission,* 2nd Internat. Pharmacol. Meeting, Prague. Pergamon Press, Oxford

[187] HOLMSTEDT B. and SJÖQVIST F. (1959) *Acta physiol scand.* **47,** 284

[189] GARDINER J. E., HELLMANN K. and THOMPSON J. W. (1962) *J. Physiol.* (Lond.) **163,** 436

[190] BURN J. H. and PHILPOT F. J. (1953) *Brit. J. Pharmacol.* **8,** 248

[191] ERÄNKÖ O. (1966) *Pharmacol. Rev.* **18,** 353

[192] BOWMAN W. C., CALLINGHAM B. A. and CUTHBERT A. W. (1964) *Brit. J. Pharmacol.* **22,** 558

[193] CARLSSON A. and WALDECK B. (1965) *J. Pharm. Pharmacol.* **17,** 243

[194] WOLNER E. (1965) Naunyn-Schmiedeberg's *Arch. exp. Path. u. Pharmakol.* **250,** 437

[198] NG KEVIN K. F. (1966) *J. Physiol.* (Lond.), **182,** 233

[199] MARRAZZI, A. (1939) *J. Pharmacol. exp. Ther.* **65,** 395

[200] BÜLBRING, E. and BURN, J. H. (1942) *J. Physiol* (Lond.) **101,** 289

[201] BÜLBRING, E. (1944) *J. Physiol.* (Lond.) **103,** 55

[202] BÜLBRING, E. and BURN, J. H. (1942) *J. Physiol.* (Lond.) **101**, 224

[203] BOWMAN, W. C. and RAPER, C. (1964) *Brit. J. Pharmacol.* **23**, 184

[204] BLASCHKO, H. (1939) *J. Physiol.* (Lond.) **96**, 50P

[205] HOLTZ, P. (1939) *Naturwissenschaften*, **27**, 724

[206] DEMIS, D. J., BLASCHKO, H. and WELCH, A. D. (1955) *J. Pharmacol. exp. Ther.* **113**, 14

[207] BÜLBRING, E. (1960) *Adrenergic Mechanisms*, p. 275, London, J. and A. Churchill Ltd.

[208] BUEDING, E. and BÜLBRING, E. (1967) *Ann. N.Y. Acad. Sci.* **139**, 758

[209] SUTHERLAND, E. and RALL, T. W. (1960) *Pharmacol. Rev.* **12**, 265

[210] SUTHERLAND, E. and ROBISON, G. A. (1966) *Pharmacol. Rev.* **18**, 145

[211] ORLOFF, J. and HANDLER, J. S. (1964) *Amer. J. Med.* **36**, 686

[212] NORTHROP, G. and PARKS, R. E. (1964) *J. Pharmacol. exp. Ther.* **145**, 135

[213] BITENSKY, M. W. and BURSTEIN, S. R. (1965) *Nature*, **208**, 1282

[214] ROBISON, G. A., BUTCHER, R. W. and SUTHERLAND, E. (1967) *Ann. N.Y. Acad. Sci.* **139**, 703

[215] BRECKENRIDGE, B. M., BURN, J. H. and MATSCHINSKY, F. (1967) *Proc. Nat. Acad. Sci.*

[216] BÜLBRING, E., GOODFORD, P. J. and SETEKLEIV, J. (1966) *Brit. J. Pharmacol.* **28**, 296

[217] JENKINSON, D. H. and MORTON, I. K. M. (1967) *Ann. N.Y. Acad. Sci.* **139**, 762

[218] DALE, H. H. (1906) *J. Physiol.* (Lond.) **34**, 163

[219] POWELL, C. E. and SLATER, I. H. (1958) *J. Pharmacol. exp. Ther.* **122**, 480

[220] BOYD, H., CHANG, V. and RAND, M. J. (1960) *Brit. J. Pharmacol.* **15**, 525

[221] BURN, J. H. and GIBBONS, W. R. (1964) *Brit. J. Pharmacol.* **22**, 527.

[222] IVERSEN, L. L. (1965) *Brit. J. Pharmacol.* **25**, 18

[223] KOPIN, I. J., FISCHER, J. E., MUSACCHIO, J. and HORST, W. D. (1964) *Proc. Nat. Acad. Sci., U.S.A.* **52**, 716

[224] KOELLE, G. B. (1961) *Nature*, **190**, 208

[225] DE GROAT, W. C. and VOLLE, R. L. (1966) *J. Pharmacol. exp. Ther.* **154**, 1

[226] ARMITAGE, A. K., MILTON, A. S. and MORRISON, C. F. (1966) *Brit. J. Pharmacol.* **27**, 33

[227] ARMITAGE, A. K. and HALL, G. H. (1967) *Nature*, **214**, 977

[228] MORRISON, C. F. and ARMITAGE, A. K. (1967) *Ann. N.Y. Acad. Sci.* **142**, 268

[229] BOVET, D. (1965) *Tobacco alkaloids and related compounds.* Ed. U.S. v. Euler, p. 125

[230] CROUT, J. R. (1964) Naunyn-Schmiedeberg's *Arch. exp. Path. Pharmakol.* **248**, 85

[231] IVERSEN, L. L. (1967) *The uptake and storage of noradrenaline in sympathetic nerves.* Chapter 9. Cambridge University Press

[232] RICHARDSON, J. A. and WOODS, E. F. (1959) *Proc. Soc. exp. Biol. Med.* **100**, 149

[233] CABRERA, R., TORRANCE, R. W. and VIVEROS, H. (1966) *Brit. J. Pharmacol.* **27**, 51

[234] FISCHER, J. E., WEISE, V. K. and KOPIN, I. J. (1966) *J. Pharmacol. exp. Ther.* **153**, 523

[235] BOYD, J. D. (1960) *Adrenergic Mechanisms,* p. 63. London, J. and A. Churchill Ltd.

[236] BURN, J. H. and WELSH, F. (1967) *Brit. J. Pharmocol.* **31**, 74.

[237] DE LA LANDE, I. S. and RAND, M. J. (1966) *Aust. J. exp. Biol. med. Sci.* **43**, 639

[238] RAND, M. J. and WILSON, J. (1967) *Eur. J. Pharmacol.* **1**, 210

[239] HOLTON, P. and ING, H. R. (1949) *Brit. J. Pharmacol.* **4**, 190

[240] GREEN, A. F. and HUGHES, R. (1966) *Brit. J. Pharmacol.* **27**, 164

[241] BOULLIN, D. J., COSTA, E. and BRODIE, B. B. (1966) *Life Sciences,* **5**, 803

[242] VINCENZI, F. F. and WEST, T. C. (1965) *Brit. J. Pharmacol.* **24**, 773.

[243] VINCENZI, F. F. (1967) *Nature,* **213**, 394

[244] BURN, J. H., PHILPOT, F. J. and TRENDELENBURG, U. (1954) *Brit. J. Pharmacol.* **9**, 423

[245] HUKOVIĆ, S. (1966) *Brit. J. Pharmacol.* **28**, 273

[246] ARMITAGE, A. K. and BURN, J. H. (1967) *Brit. J. Pharmacol.* **29**, 218.

[247] YOUNG, J. Z. (1936) *Proc. Roy. Soc.* Ser. B, **120**, 303

[248] BURNSTOCK, G. (1958) *Brit. J. Pharmacol.* **13**, 216

[249] BOATMAN, D. L., SHAFFER, R. A., DIXON, R. L. and BRODY, M. J. (1965) *J. Clin. Invest.* **44**, 241

[255] GLOWINSKI, J., AXELROD, J., KOPIN, I. J. and WURTMAN, R. J. (1964) *J. Pharmacol. exp. Ther.* **146**, 48

[256] RICHARDSON, K. C. (1966) *Nature* (Lond.) **210**, 756

[257] TRANZER, J. P. and THOENEN, H. (1967) *Experientia,* **23**, 123

[258] KOELLE, G. B. (1965) Second International Pharmacological Meeting. Vol. 3. *Pharmacology of Cholinergic and Adrenergic Transmission,* p. 29. Pergamon Press, London

[259] BURN, J. H. and NG, KEVIN K. F. (1965) *Brit. J. Pharmacol.* **24**, 675

[260] McGiff, J. C., Burns, R. B. P. and Blumenthal, M. R. (1967) *Circulation Res.* **20**, 616

[261] Finkleman, B. (1930) *J. Physiol.* (Lond.) 70, 145

[262] Blinks, J. R. (1966) *J. Pharmocol. exp. Ther.* **151**, 221

[263] Levi-Montalcini, R. and Angeletti, P. U. (1966) *Pharmocol. Rev.* **18**, 619

[264] Vogt, M. (1964) *Nature, Lond.* **204**, 1315

[265] Renshaw, R. R., Green, D. and Ziff, M. (1938) *J. Pharmocol. exp. Ther.* **62**, 430

[266] Malik, K. U. and Ling, G. M. (1969) *Circulation Res.* **25**, 1

[267] Malik, K. U. and Ling, G. M. (1969) *J. Pharm. Pharmacol.* **21**, 514

[268] Ambache, N., Perry, W. L. M. and Robertson, P. A. (1956) *Brit. J. Pharmacol.* **11**, 442

[269] Reinert, H. (1960) *Adrenergic Mechanisms*, p. 373. London, J. and A. Churchill Ltd.

[270] Muscholl, E. and Maitre, L. (1963) *Experientia*, **19**, 658

[271] Kopin, I. J. (1968) *Adrenergic Neurotransmission*, Ciba Foundation Study Group No. 33. p. 95. London, J. and A. Churchill Ltd.

[272] Carr, L. A. and Moore, K. E. (1969) *Science*, **164**, 322

[273] Philippu, A., Heyd, G. and Burger, A. (1970) *Europ. J. Pharmacol.* **9**, 52

[274] Burn, J. H. and Malik, K. U. (1970) *J. Physiol.* (Lond.) **208**, 82P

[275] Curtis, D. R., Duggan, A. W., Felix, D., and Johnstone, G. A. R. (1970) *Nature* (Lond.) **226**, 1222

[276] Burn, J. H. and Gibbons, W. R. (1965) *J. Physiol.* (Lond.) **181**, 214

[277] Eccleston, D., Randić, M., Roberts, M. H. T. and Straughan, D. W. (1969) *Metabolism of Amines in the Brain*, p. 29. London, Macmillan

[278] Jouvet, M. and Renault, J. (1966) *Compt. rend. Séanc. Soc. Biol.* **160**, 1461

[279] Vogt, M. (1969) *Brit. J. Pharmacol.* **37**, 325

[280] Feldberg, W. and Myers, R. D. (1964) *J. Physiol.* (Lond.) **173**, 226

[281] Bülbring, E. and Gershon, M. D. (1967) *J. Physiol.* (Lond.) **192**, 823

[282] Kottegoda, S. R. (1969) *J. Physiol.* (Lond.) **200**, 687

[283] Quay, W. B. and Halevy, A. (1962) *Physiol. Zool.* **35**, 1

[284] Bertler, Å., Falck, B. and Owman, C. (1964) *Acta physiol. scand.* Suppl. 239, p. 1

[285] Lichtensteiger, W., Mutzner, U. and Langemann, H. (1967) *J. Neurochem.* **14**, 489

[286] Zweig, M. and Axelrod, J. (1969) *J. Neurobiol.* **1**, 87

[287] BORN, G. V. R. and GILLSON, R. E. (1959) *J. Physiol.* (Lond.) **146,** 472

[288] HAEUSLER, G., THOENEN, H., HAEFELY, W. and HUERLIMANN, A. (1968) Naunyn-Schmiedeberg's *Arch. Pharmak. exp. Path.* **261,** 389

[289] V. EULER, U. S. (1935) *Klin. Wschr.* **14,** 1182

[290] AMBACHE, N. (1957) *J. Physiol.* (Lond.) **135,** 114

[291] HILTON, S. M. and LEWIS, G. P. (1956) *J. Physiol.* (Lond.) **134,** 471

[292] GOODWIN, L. G. and RICHARDS, W. H. G. (1960) *Brit. J. Pharmacol.* **15,** 152

[293] MELMON, K. L. and CLINE, M. J. (1967) *Nature* (Lond.) **213,** 90

[294] HARRIS, G. W. and NAFTOLIN, F. (1970) *Brit. Med. Bull.* **26,** 3

[295] CARLSSON, A., FALCK, B., HILLARP, N. A. and TORP, A. (1962) *Acta physiol. scand.* **54,** 385

[296] MCGREGOR, D. D. (1965) *J. Physiol.* (Lond.) **177,** 21

[297] FOLKOW, B. (1955) *Physiol. Rev.* **35,** 629

[298] MALIK, K. U. (1969) *J. Pharm. Pharmacol.* **21,** 472

[299] MALIK, K. U. and LING, G. M. (1969) *Circulation Res.* **25,** 1-9

[300] BÜLBRING, E. (1946) *Brit. J. Pharmacol.* **1,** 38, Fig. 12

[301] LINDMAR, R., LOFFELHOLZ, K. and MUSCHOLL, E. (1968) *Brit. J. Pharmacol.* **32,** 280

[302] MALIK, K. U. (1970) *Circulation Res.* **27,** 647–656

[303] EHINGER, B. and FALCK, B. (1965) *Life Sci.* **4,** 2097

[304] EHINGER, B., FALCK, B. and SPORRONG (1970) *Zeitschr. f. Zellforschung,* **107,** 508

[305] WATERSON, J. G., HUME, W. R. and DE LA LANDE, I. S. (1970) *J. Histochem. and Cytochem.* **18,** 211

[306] ARMITAGE, A. K., HALL, G. H. and MORRISON, C. F. (1968) *Nature* (Lond.) **217,** 331

[307] SPELLER, P. J. and STREETEN, D. H. P. (1964) *Metabolism* **13,** 453

INDEX

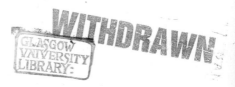